I0510973

MEDICAID AT 50: STRENGTHENING AND SUSTAINING THE PROGRAM

HEARING

BEFORE THE

SUBCOMMITTEE ON HEALTH

OF THE

COMMITTEE ON ENERGY AND COMMERCE

HOUSE OF REPRESENTATIVES

ONE HUNDRED FOURTEENTH CONGRESS

FIRST SESSION

JULY 8, 2015

Serial No. 114–63

Printed for the use of the Committee on Energy and Commerce

energycommerce.house.gov

U.S. GOVERNMENT PUBLISHING OFFICE

97–774 PDF   WASHINGTON : 2016

For sale by the Superintendent of Documents, U.S. Government Publishing Office
Internet: bookstore.gpo.gov   Phone: toll free (866) 512–1800; DC area (202) 512–1800
Fax: (202) 512–2104   Mail: Stop IDCC, Washington, DC 20402–0001

COMMITTEE ON ENERGY AND COMMERCE

FRED UPTON, Michigan
Chairman

JOE BARTON, Texas
Chairman Emeritus
ED WHITFIELD, Kentucky
JOHN SHIMKUS, Illinois
JOSEPH R. PITTS, Pennsylvania
GREG WALDEN, Oregon
TIM MURPHY, Pennsylvania
MICHAEL C. BURGESS, Texas
MARSHA BLACKBURN, Tennessee
Vice Chairman
STEVE SCALISE, Louisiana
ROBERT E. LATTA, Ohio
CATHY McMORRIS RODGERS, Washington
GREGG HARPER, Mississippi
LEONARD LANCE, New Jersey
BRETT GUTHRIE, Kentucky
PETE OLSON, Texas
DAVID B. McKINLEY, West Virginia
MIKE POMPEO, Kansas
ADAM KINZINGER, Illinois
H. MORGAN GRIFFITH, Virginia
GUS M. BILIRAKIS, Florida
BILL JOHNSON, Ohio
BILLY LONG, Missouri
RENEE L. ELLMERS, North Carolina
LARRY BUCSHON, Indiana
BILL FLORES, Texas
SUSAN W. BROOKS, Indiana
MARKWAYNE MULLIN, Oklahoma
RICHARD HUDSON, North Carolina
CHRIS COLLINS, New York
KEVIN CRAMER, North Dakota

FRANK PALLONE, Jr., New Jersey
Ranking Member
BOBBY L. RUSH, Illinois
ANNA G. ESHOO, California
ELIOT L. ENGEL, New York
GENE GREEN, Texas
DIANA DeGETTE, Colorado
LOIS CAPPS, California
MICHAEL F. DOYLE, Pennsylvania
JANICE D. SCHAKOWSKY, Illinois
G.K. BUTTERFIELD, North Carolina
DORIS O. MATSUI, California
KATHY CASTOR, Florida
JOHN P. SARBANES, Maryland
JERRY McNERNEY, California
PETER WELCH, Vermont
BEN RAY LUJAN, New Mexico
PAUL TONKO, New York
JOHN A. YARMUTH, Kentucky
YVETTE D. CLARKE, New York
DAVID LOEBSACK, Iowa
KURT SCHRADER, Oregon
JOSEPH P. KENNEDY, III, Massachusetts
TONY CARDENAS, California7

SUBCOMMITTEE ON HEALTH

JOSEPH R. PITTS, Pennsylvania
Chairman

BRETT GUTHRIE, Kentucky
Vice Chairman
ED WHITFIELD, Kentucky
JOHN SHIMKUS, Illinois
TIM MURPHY, Pennsylvania
MICHAEL C. BURGESS, Texas
MARSHA BLACKBURN, Tennessee
CATHY McMORRIS RODGERS, Washington
LEONARD LANCE, New Jersey
H. MORGAN GRIFFITH, Virginia
GUS M. BILIRAKIS, Florida
BILLY LONG, Missouri
RENEE L. ELLMERS, North Carolina
LARRY BUCSHON, Indiana
SUSAN W. BROOKS, Indiana
CHRIS COLLINS, New York
JOE BARTON, Texas
FRED UPTON, Michigan *(ex officio)*

GENE GREEN, Texas
Ranking Member
ELIOT L. ENGEL, New York
LOIS CAPPS, California
JANICE D. SCHAKOWSKY, Illinois
G.K. BUTTERFIELD, North Carolina
KATHY CASTOR, Florida
JOHN P. SARBANES, Maryland
DORIS O. MATSUI, California
BEN RAY LUJAN, New Mexico
KURT SCHRADER, Oregon
JOSEPH P. KENNEDY, III, Massachusetts
TONY CARDENAS, California
FRANK PALLONE, Jr., New Jersey *(ex officio)*

C O N T E N T S

---

[1] Ms. Wachino's response to submitted questions for the record has been retained in committee files and also is available at *http://docs.house.gov/meetings/IF/IF14/20150708/103717/HHRG-114-IF14-Wstate-WachinoV-20150708-SD002.pdf*.

[2] Ms. Yocom and Ms. Iritani provided a joint response to submitted questions for the record.

[3] Ms. Iritani submitted a joint statement for the record with Ms. Yocom but did not submit an oral statement.

MEDICAID AT 50: STRENGTHENING AND SUSTAINING THE PROGRAM

WEDNESDAY, JULY 8, 2015

House of Representatives,
Subcommittee on Health,
Committee on Energy and Commerce,
Washington, DC.

The subcommittee met, pursuant to call, at 10:14 a.m., in room 2322 of the Rayburn House Office Building, Hon. Joe Pitts (chairman of the subcommittee) presiding.

Members present: Representatives Pitts, Guthrie, Barton, Whitfield, Shimkus, Murphy, Burgess, Blackburn, Lance, Griffith, Bilirakis, Long, Ellmers, Brooks, Collins, Green, Capps, Schakowsky, Butterfield, Castor, Sarbanes, Matsui, Luján, Schrader, Kennedy, Cárdenas, and Pallone (ex officio).

Staff present: Graham Pittman, Legislative Clerk; David Redl, Chief Counsel, Communications and Technology; Michelle Rosenberg, GAO Detailee, Health; Krista Rosenthall, Counsel to Chairman Emeritus; Heidi Stirrup, Policy Coordinator, Health; Josh Trent, Professional Staff Member, Health; Traci Vitek, Detailee, Health; Christine Brennan, Democratic Press Secretary; Jeff Carroll, Democratic Staff Director; Tiffany Guarascio, Democratic Deputy Staff Director and Chief Health Advisor; Una Lee, Democratic Chief Oversight Counsel; Rachel Pryor, Democratic Health Policy Advisor; and Samantha Satchell, Democratic Policy Analyst.

Mr. PITTS. Good morning, and welcome to this hearing, entitled Medicaid at 50: Strengthening and Sustaining the Program. Subcommittee will come to order. Chairman will recognize himself for an opening statement.

OPENING STATEMENT OF HON. JOSEPH R. PITTS, A REPRESENTATIVE IN CONGRESS FROM THE COMMONWEALTH OF PENNSYLVANIA

At the end of this month, Medicaid will turn 50 years old. It was created as a joint Federal/State program to provide healthcare coverage to certain categories of low-income Americans. But today Medicaid is now the largest health insurance program in the world. Now more than 70 million Americans are covered by Medicaid, which is more than are covered by Medicare. No doubt Medicaid is a critical lifeline for some of our Nation's most vulnerable patients. Medicaid provides health care for children, pregnant mothers, the elderly, the blind, and the disabled. It is safe to say that every member of this committee wants to see a strong safety net program that protects the most vulnerable, regardless of how they feel about its recent expansion.

But, as we all know, the current trajectory of Medicaid spending is problematic. In the next decade, program outlays are set to double. That means that, in a decade, Medicaid is going to cost Federal taxpayers what Medicare costs today. And that is not even counting the fact that the Medicaid program is already the fastest growing spending item in most State budgets. So, without Congressional intervention, Medicaid will continue to consume a larger and larger portion of Federal and State spending. This is not ideology. This is arithmetic. According to CBO data, by 2030, the entire Federal budget will be consumed with spending on mandatory entitlements and service on the debt.

And this is not only a budgetary problem, though such levels of spending would crowd out funding for other important Federal and State policy priorities. This is also not only a fiscal problem, though CBO has warned that running up our national credit card could trigger financial crisis. Perhaps most importantly, this spending trajectory threatens the quality and access of care for the millions of vulnerable patients who depend on Medicaid.

But reaching the breaking point is entirely preventable. Policymaking is about setting priorities and making choices, and that is why, and many of my colleagues were dismayed by some of what we learned at a recent Health Subcommittee hearing regarding some of the projects funded through waivers. With budgets growing, is it too radical to suggest we simply prioritize needed medical care over lower priority projects?

Since 2003 Medicaid has been designated a high risk program by the GAO because of its size, growth, diversity programs, concerns about gaps, and fiscal oversight. More than a decade later, these issues are amplified by recent changes to the program. Our aging population will also increase demands on the program. But today Federal oversight of the program is more imperative than ever.

Each administration has a responsibility, with Congress, to ensure that taxpayer dollars used for Medicaid are spent in a manner that helps our neediest citizens. Thus, I am pleased that we have a distinguished panel of witnesses today to help inform us on the challenges facing Medicaid in the coming decade. I am especially pleased that CMS, who was unable to attend—to join us for our recent hearing is here today, along with GAO and MACPAC.

In order to preserve and strengthen this vital safety net program for the most vulnerable, I believe that Congress will be increasingly forced to take steps to modernize the Medicaid program. So we are eager to hear our witnesses' recommendations for ideas, and any efforts underway to enhance Medicaid program efficiency, reduce program costs, and improve quality.

[The prepared statement of Mr. Pitts follows:]

PREPARED STATEMENT OF HON. JOSEPH R. PITTS

At the end of this month, Medicaid will turn 50 years old. It was created as a joint Federal/State program to provide healthcare coverage to certain categories of low-income Americans.

But today, Medicaid is now the largest health insurance program in the world. Now more than 70 million Americans are covered by Medicaid—which is more than are covered by Medicare.

No doubt, Medicaid is a critical lifeline for some of our Nation's most vulnerable patients. Medicaid provides health care for children, pregnant mothers, the elderly, the blind, and the disabled. It is safe to say that every member of this committee wants to see a strong safety net program that protects the most vulnerable—regardless of how they feel about its recent expansion.

But as we all know, the current trajectory of Medicaid spending is problematic. In the next decade, program outlays are set to double. That means that in a decade, Medicaid is going to cost Federal taxpayers what Medicare costs today—and that's not even counting the fact that the Medicaid program is already the fastest growing spending item in most State budgets.

So, without Congressional intervention, Medicaid will continue to consume a larger and larger portion of Federal and State spending. This is not ideology, this is arithmetic. According to CBO data, by 2030, the entire Federal budget will be consumed with spending on mandatory entitlements and service on the debt.

This is not only a budgetary problem—though such levels of spending would crowd out funding for other important Federal and State policy priorities. This is also not only a fiscal problem—though CBO has warned that running up our national credit card could trigger another financial crisis. Perhaps most importantly, this spending trajectory threatens the quality and access of care for the millions of vulnerable patients who depend on Medicaid.

But reaching the breaking point is entirely preventable. Policy-making is about setting priorities and making choices.

That's why I and many of my colleagues were dismayed by some of what we learned at a recent Health Subcommittee hearing regarding some of the projects funded through waivers. With budgets growing, is it too radical to suggest we simply prioritize needed medical care, over lower-priority projects?

Since 2003, Medicaid has been designated a high-risk program by the GAO because of its size, growth, diversity of programs, and concerns about gaps in fiscal oversight. More than a decade later, these issues are amplified by recent changes to the program. Our aging population will also increase demands on the program. But today, Federal oversight of the program is more imperative than ever. Each administration has a responsibility, with Congress, to ensure that taxpayer dollars used for Medicaid are spent in a manner that helps our neediest citizens.

Thus, I am pleased that we have a distinguished panel of witnesses today to help inform us on the challenges facing Medicaid in the coming decade. I am especially pleased that CMS, who was unable to join us for our recent hearing, is here today, along with GAO and MACPAC.

In order to preserve and strengthen this vital safety net program for the most vulnerable, I believe that Congress will be increasingly forced to take steps to modernize the Medicaid program. So we are eager to hear our witnesses' recommendations for ideas and any efforts underway to enhance Medicaid program efficiency, reduce program costs, and improve quality.

Mr. PITTS. And, with that, I yield back and recognize the ranking member, Mr. Green, 5 minutes for his opening statement.

OPENING STATEMENT OF HON. GENE GREEN, A REPRESENTATIVE IN CONGRESS FROM THE STATE OF TEXAS

Mr. GREEN. Thank you, Mr. Chairman, for holding the hearings, and I too want to welcome our panel. It is not very often that we get an all-female panel. I appreciate you all being here.

The Medicaid program has served as a critical safety net for the American public since its creation in 1965, 50 years ago this month. Today, over 70 million low-income Americans rely on Medicaid for comprehensive and affordable health insurance. It is a lifeline for millions of children, pregnant women, people with disabilities, seniors, and low-income adults. Medicaid covers more than one in three children, pays for nearly half of all births, accounts for more than 40 percent of the Nation's total costs for long-term care. One in seven Medicare beneficiaries are also Medicaid beneficiaries. The Medicaid accounts for a quarter of behavioral healthcare services.

4

The Affordable Care Act expanded coverage, made improvements to promote program integrity, transparency, and advanced delivery system reform. Since the enactment of the Affordable Care Act, the overall rate of healthcare spending growth has slowed, reducing projected growth in Medicaid programs by hundreds of billions of dollars, according to the Congressional Budget Office. This is primarily due to lower than expected growth in costs per Medicaid enrollee.

The need to address the growth of healthcare spending is an issue, we all agree. We must remain committed to building on the progress made by the ACA in ensuring patients have access to quality, affordable care, and that we are getting the best value for our healthcare dollars. Medicaid is an extremely efficient program, covering the average enrollee at a lower cost than most comprehensive benefits, and significantly lower cost sharing then private insurance. 95 percent of Medicaid beneficiaries report having a regular source of health care, a medical home in today's terms, which they consistently rate as highly as private insurance.

As we examine ways to further strengthen and improve the program, we need to advance policies that better leverage dollars to pay for value, promote efficiency and transparency, and advance delivery system reforms, and extend innovative strategies within Medicaid, and across the healthcare system. For example, one improvement would be for the Centers of Medicaid and—Medicare and Medicaid Services to finalize the agency's proposed regulation that would better enforce the Medicaid's equal access provision. This provision ensures that care and services are available to Medicaid enrollees, and that providers are paid a fair Medicaid reimbursement rate.

Another one would be the require 12 month continuous enrollment—eligible Medicaid and CHIP beneficiaries to address the issue of the churn, a concept that MACPAC has supported in several reports to Congress. Churn is bad for patients, providers, and health plans, and wastes taxpayers' dollars. I worked with my colleague Joe Barton for several Congresses on this legislation—on this issue, and I thank him for his leadership, on behalf of low-income Americans.

Today we look at a broad—look at the Medicaid system, the past, present, and future. Throughout its 50 year history, Medicaid has served as an adaptable, efficient program that meets the healthcare needs of millions of Americans. I want to thank our witnesses again for their ongoing efforts and recommendations for additional ways to advance the program. I look forward to working with my colleagues on the committee to strengthen the program in key areas, including the enrollment process, delivery system reforms, managed care, data collection, and behavioral health.

[The prepared statement of Mr. Green follows:]

PREPARED STATEMENT OF HON. GENE GREEN

Thank you, Mr. Chairman, for holding this hearing.

The Medicaid program has served as a critical safety net for the American public since its creation in 1965, 50 years ago this month.

Today, over 70 million low-income Americans rely on Medicaid for comprehensive, affordable health insurance.

It is a lifeline for millions of children, pregnant women, people with disabilities, seniors, and low-income adults.

Medicaid covers more than 1 in 3 children, pays for nearly half of all births, and accounts for more than 40 percent of the Nation's total costs for long-term care.

One in seven Medicare beneficiaries is also a Medicaid beneficiary, and Medicaid accounts for a quarter of all behavioral health services.

The Affordable Care Act expanded coverage, made improvements to promote program integrity and transparency, and advanced delivery system reform.

Since the enactment of the Affordable Care Act, the overall rate of healthcare spending growth has slowed, reducing projected growth in the Medicaid programs by hundreds of billions of dollars according to the Congressional Budget Office.

This is primarily due to lower than expected growth in costs per Medicaid enrollee.

The need to address the growth of healthcare spending is an issue on which we all agree.

We must remain committed to building on the progress made by the ACA, ensuring patients have access to quality, affordable care, and that we are getting the best value for our healthcare dollars.

Medicaid is an extremely efficient program, covering the average enrollee at a lower cost with more comprehensive benefits and significantly lower cost-sharing than private insurance.

Ninety-five percent of Medicaid beneficiaries report having a regular source of health care, which they consistently rate as highly as private insurance.

As we examine ways to further strength and improve the program, we need to advance policies that better leverage dollars to pay for value, promote efficacy and transparency, advance delivery system reforms, and extend innovative strategies within Medicaid and across the healthcare system.

For example, one improvement would be for the Centers for Medicare and Medicaid Services (CMS) to finalize the agency's proposed regulation that would better enforce the Medicaid's equal access provision.

This provision ensures that care and services are available to Medicaid enrollees, and that providers are paid a fair Medicaid reimbursement rate.

Another would be to require 12-month continuous enrollment for eligible Medicaid and CHIP beneficiaries to address the issue of "churn," a concept MACPAC has supported in several reports to Congress.

Churn is bad for patients, providers, and health plans, and wastes taxpayer dollars.

I have worked with my colleague, Joe Barton, for several Congresses on legislation on this issue, and I thank him for his leadership on behalf of low-income Americans.

Today, we will take a broad look at the Medicaid system: its past, present, and future.

Throughout its 50-year history, Medicaid has served as an adaptable, efficient program that meets the healthcare needs of millions of Americans.

I want to thank our witnesses for their on-going efforts and recommendations for additional ways to advance of the program.

I look forward to working with my colleagues on the committee to strengthen the program in key areas, including the enrollment process, delivery system reforms and managed care, data collection, and behavioral health.

Thank you, and I yield the balance of my time to my colleague from California, Congresswoman Matsui.

Mr. GREEN. With that, Mr. Chairman, I would like to yield the balance of my time to my colleague from California, Congresswoman Matsui.

Ms. MATSUI. Thank you very much for yielding to me, and I would like to welcome our witnesses here today also. This year, as we know, we celebrate the 50th anniversary of both the Medicare and Medicaid programs, essential programs for the security of our Nation's seniors, people with disabilities, children, and families. The Affordable Care Act took vital steps to reforming our healthcare system by increasing coverage and moving toward rewarding value, instead of volume. We know the ACA made improvements in the private insurance market, and it also made improvements for public programs like Medicaid. Now is the time that we need to build upon those improvements, and keep the momentum going for our healthcare system, and for the millions that rely on Medicaid as an important safety net.

Thank you, and I look forward to hearing from our witnesses today, and I yield time to whoever needs it.

Mr. GREEN. Anyone else want 40 seconds, or—I yield back.

Mr. PITTS. The gentleman yields back, and now the Chair recognizes the ranking member of the full committee, Mr. Pallone, 5 minutes for an opening statement.

OPENING STATEMENT OF HON. FRANK PALLONE, JR., A REPRESENTATIVE IN CONGRESS FROM THE STATE OF NEW JERSEY

Mr. PALLONE. Thank you, Mr. Chairman. I just want to say, obviously, this is a very important topic. Medicaid's 50 years of efficient, comprehensive, and sometimes life-saving health coverage of our most vulnerable populations is certainly something that is crucial. A fiber, you know, basic fabric of our healthcare system.

As Members of Congress, I believe the Government can help all Americans succeed, including seniors and low-income families, and improving and strengthening Medicaid for generations to come continues to be a primary goal. Medicaid provides more than one in three children with a chance at a healthy start in life, and one in seven Medicare seniors are also actually Medicaid seniors. In fact, the overwhelming majority of the 71 million current Medicaid beneficiaries are children, the elderly, the disabled, and pregnant women.

We often talk about Medicaid as an entitlement program, though I don't believe this is true—a true reflection of the program. Medicaid is a bedrock safety net that ensures all Americans have protection against the negative economic effects that undisputedly come with lack of health coverage. Medicaid's inherent structure was designed to ensure that health coverage will be there for those who need it, when times are hard, jobs are lost, or accidents strike. And the fundamental tenet of the program is that it can expand and contract according to need. In fact, Medicaid was first proposed as part of a set of economic policies by President Truman.

And the Affordable Care Act built on these same goals by strengthening Medicaid and expanding its coverage, and States that have expanded Medicaid have already realized significant qualitative and economic benefits as uncompensated care rates drop, and more people gain coverage. Meanwhile, Medicaid coverage lowers financial barriers to healthcare access, increases use of preventative care, and improves health outcomes. In addition, States have been successful in managing their Medicaid programs through broad latitude and flexibility to ensure access to critical healthcare services for their populations at low cost.

No program is perfect. For instance, I believe that we need to remain vigilant on access to specialty and dental care, and we continue to refine transparency and evaluation of Medicaid waivers, and ensure that Medicaid is successfully integrated with Medicare in the health insurance marketplaces. We should think more about how to advance some of the innovations in delivery systems reform.

The Medicaid program has some of our best successes, with some of the toughest to treat populations.

Mr. Chairman, I hope to hear—to not hear more today of the same assaults on the Affordable Care Act or Medicaid. Inaccurate and ideological representation of what Medicaid is and who it serves I think are outdated. Instead, I believe that there are many policy areas in Medicaid where members on both the Democrat and Republican sides could share an interest, and I look forward to learning about ways that Congress can help to build on an already strong Medicaid program, refining and modernizing this critical safety net for the next 50 years and beyond.

[The prepared statement of Mr. Pallone follows:]

PREPARED STATEMENT OF HON. FRANK PALLONE, JR.

Thank you, Mr. Chairman, for convening a hearing on this timely and important topic—Medicaid's 50 years of efficient, comprehensive, and sometimes lifesaving, health coverage of our most vulnerable populations. As a Member of Congress, I believe that Government can help all Americans succeed, including seniors and low-income families, and improving and strengthening Medicaid for generations to come continues to be a primary goal of mine.

Medicaid provides more than 1 in 3 children with a chance at a healthy start in life. And 1 in 7 Medicare seniors are actually also Medicaid seniors. In fact, the overwhelming majority of the 71 million current Medicaid beneficiaries are children, the elderly, the disabled and pregnant women.

We often talk about Medicaid as an entitlement program. Though I don't believe this is a true reflection of the program. Medicaid is a bedrock safety net that ensures all Americans have protection against the negative economic effects that undisputedly come with lack of health coverage. Medicaid's inherent structure was designed to ensure that health coverage will be there for those who need it when times are hard, jobs are lost, or accident strikes. The fundamental tenet of the program is that it can expand and contract according to need. In fact, Medicaid was first proposed as part of a set of economic policies by President Truman.

And the Affordable Care Act built on those same goals, by strengthening Medicaid and expanding its coverage. States that have expanded Medicaid have already realized significant qualitative and economic benefits as uncompensated care rates drop and more people gain coverage. Meanwhile, Medicaid coverage lowers financial barriers to healthcare access, increases use of preventative care, and improves health outcomes.

In addition, States have been successful in managing their Medicaid programs through broad latitude and flexibility to ensure access to critical healthcare services for their own populations at low costs.

No program is perfect; For instance, I believe that we need to remain vigilant on access to specialty and dental care, continue to refine transparency and evaluation of Medicaid waivers, and ensure that Medicaid is successfully integrated with Medicare and the health insurance marketplaces. We should think more about how to advance some of the innovations in delivery system reform-the Medicaid program has some of our best successes, with some of the toughest-to-treat populations.

Mr. Chairman, I hope to not hear more of the same assaults on the Affordable Care Act or Medicaid today. Inaccurate and ideological representations of what Medicaid is and who it serves are tired and outdated. Instead, I believe that there are many policy areas in Medicaid where members on both sides could share an interest. I look forward to learning about ways that Congress can help to build on an already strong Medicaid program, refining and modernizing this critical safety net for the next 50 years and beyond.

Mr. PALLONE. I would like to yield the 2 minutes—or the remainder of my time to Mr. Luján.

Mr. LUJÁN. Thank you very much, Mr. Chairman and Ranking Member Pallone, for scheduling this hearing. And I am glad that we are here, coming together to reflect on the success of this program as we celebrate its 50th anniversary.

Medicaid is a critical program across the Nation, and especially in my home State of New Mexico, where we have had a 53 percent increase in enrollment since we expanded Medicaid. This represents 240,000 additional people who have gained coverage as a result of the Affordable Care Act's Medicaid expansion in New Mexico. Behind each of these statistics are real stories of New Mexicans whose lives have improved because of Medicaid. I believe deeply in Medicaid's mission of improving access to health care, better health outcomes, greater financial security, and that we have a responsibility to ensure that our constituents are not only covered, but also receive quality care.

I look forward to the testimony and discussion about how we can continue to enhance this program for the next 50 years and beyond, and I also have some very serious specific questions about New Mexico's behavioral health program, and I look forward to exploring those as well. So, Mr. Chairman, Ranking Member Pallone, I thank you for the time, and I yield back.

Mr. PITTS. Chair thanks the gentleman. As usual, all the members' written opening statements will be made part of the record. I have a UC request and would like to submit the following documents for the record: statements from 3M, the National Association of Chain Drugstores, the Infectious Disease Society of America, and U.S. Department of Health and Human Services Office of Inspector General, HHS/OIG. Without objection, so ordered.

[The information appears at the conclusion of the hearing.]

Mr. PITTS. We have one panel today, and let me introduce them in the order of their presentations. First, Vikki Wachino, Deputy Administrator, Centers for Medicare and Medicaid Services, CMS, and Director of the Center for Medicaid and CHIP services, CMS. Then Carolyn Yocom, Director, Health Care, Government Accountability Office, accompanied by Katherine Iritani, Director of Health Care, GAO. And finally, Anne Schwartz, Executive Director, Medicaid and CHIP Payment and Access Commission, MACPAC.

So thank you all for coming. Your written testimony will be made part of the record, and you will each be given 5 minutes to summarize your testimony. So, at this point, Ms. Wachino, you are recognized for 5 minutes for your summary.

STATEMENTS OF VIKKI WACHINO, DEPUTY ADMINISTRATOR AND DIRECTOR, CENTER FOR MEDICAID AND CHIP SERVICES, CENTERS FOR MEDICARE & MEDICAID SERVICES; CAROLYN L. YOCOM, DIRECTOR, HEALTH CARE, GOVERNMENT ACCOUNTABILITY OFFICE, ACCOMPANIED BY KATHERINE IRITANI, DIRECTOR, HEALTH CARE, GOVERNMENT ACCOUNTABILITY OFFICE; AND ANNE SCHWARTZ, PH.D., EXECUTIVE DIRECTOR, MEDICAID AND CHIP PAYMENT AND ACCESS COMMISSION

STATEMENT OF VIKKI WACHINO

Ms. WACHINO. Chairman Pitts, thank you. Ranking Member Green, thank you. Thank you, members of the subcommittee. I am happy to be with you here today to talk about the importance of the Medicaid program, and its success in meeting the needs of the low-income population over the past 50 years. Pleased to be joined here today by my colleagues from MACPAC and GAO, whose work helps us to continue to strengthen the program for the future.

I am Vikki Wachino, and I will introduce myself, building on the chairman's introduction, as Deputy Administrator and Director of the Center for Medicaid and CHIP Services. Since it is my first appearance here before the subcommittee, I have served in this role since April, and really look forward to working with the subcommittee going forward to make the program as strong as possible.

As you well know, Medicaid provides health insurance coverage to more than 70 million low-income Americans, and the beneficiaries we serve are children, low-income adults, people with disabilities, seniors, and pregnant women, some of America's most vulnerable populations. We work in partnership with States, and, as a partnership, both we and States have vital roles as program stewards in ensuring the program's future. Within Medicaid's structure, Medicaid provides vital financial support, and also significant flexibility within program rules that help us and States continue to improve and innovate in the program for the future.

The impact and success of Medicaid coverage is clear from the research. Just last month researchers at the Commonwealth Fund found that adults covered by Medicaid coverage continuously for a year have very high rates of obtaining regular sources of care. We also know, from research released earlier this year, that children who are covered by Medicaid or CHIP earn higher wages when they grow into adults, and those examples make both the health and the economic impact of Medicaid coverage clear.

There is a lot more we can do, though, and are doing, in our work with States to strengthen the program for its next 50 years and beyond. As many of you have noted, the Affordable Care Act gives States the opportunity to provide Medicaid coverage to low-income adults in their States, at their option, and supported by a substantially enhanced Federal matching rate. 28 States and the District of Columbia have worked with us to provide Medicaid coverage to these low-income adults, and the benefits of that expansion are clear. And we are prepared at CMS to work with every State to develop an approach to expansion that works for the State, meets its specific needs, and meets the needs of its low-income residents as we work together to close the coverage gap and insure more low-income Americans.

The need for modernization in our eligibility enrollment process was clear to us several years ago, and we have modernized it. We have made it substantially easier for people to apply using a single streamlined application, the same application that people applying for marketplace coverage use, and we have supported that with electronic verification. And as a result, States are able to make eligibility decisions that are fast, and accurate, and in close to real time.

Another major area of our focus is delivery system reform, and working with States to promote innovations that achieve better health, and better care, at lower cost. We carry that work out through a variety of mechanisms. Whether it is major delivery system reform initiatives, like Strong Start that is aimed at improving prenatal and maternal health, new authorities, like Health Homes for people with chronic conditions, new models, like the State innovation models that help States undertake multi-payer delivery system reforms, or pioneering delivery system reforms through our 1115 innovations. In addition to that, a year ago, at the recommendation of the Governors, we launched the Innovation Accelerator Program, which is designed to continue to advance in as many States as care to work with us, payment and delivery system reform.

As has been referenced, we have proposed major advances in managed care. Medicaid is no longer a fee-for-service delivery system. Managed care is the delivery system that provides care to the majority of our beneficiaries, and we want to maximize its potential to ensure coordination and quality of care. Our regulations had not been updated in more than a decade, and in May we proposed to update them to strengthen quality, accountability, transparency, the beneficiary experience, and also to align our roles with those that work in Medicare Advantage and in the private market, and that rule is out for public comment now.

We have been substantially advancing the ability of fragile seniors and people with disabilities to live in their communities and to self-direct their care. And underpinning all of these improvements are a commitment to program integrity that we have advanced over the past 5 years, and that span a range of mechanisms from reviewing States' program integrity programs to ensure that they are strong, to ensuring that States, and we, dedicate our resources and coordinate our resources to screen out high risk providers.

With that I will conclude, and again thank the subcommittee for your interest in the Medicaid program, and to state once again how much I am looking forward to working with each of you.

[The prepared statement of Ms. Wachino follows:]

STATEMENT OF

VIKKI WACHINO

DEPUTY ADMINISTRATOR AND DIRECTOR,
CENTER FOR MEDICAID AND CHIP SERVICES
CENTERS FOR MEDICARE & MEDICAID SERVICES

ON

MEDICAID AT 50: STRENGTHENING AND SUSTAINING THE PROGRAM

BEFORE THE

U.S. HOUSE COMMITTEE ON ENERGY & COMMERCE
SUBCOMMITTEE ON HEALTH

JULY 8, 2015

U.S. House Committee on Energy & Commerce
Subcommittee on Health
Medicaid at 50: Strengthening and Sustaining the Program
July 8, 2015

Chairman Pitts, Ranking Member Green, and members of the Subcommittee, thank you for the invitation and the opportunity to discuss the importance of the Medicaid program, reflect on some of its achievements over the past 50 years, and discuss the Centers for Medicare & Medicaid Services' (CMS') work with states in key areas such as broadening access to coverage, strengthening the quality of care through payment and delivery system reforms, and enhancing the program so that it meets the needs of our beneficiaries most effectively.

The Medicaid program provides health insurance coverage for more than 70 million Americans, playing a particularly important role in providing coverage for low-income children, adults, pregnant women, people with disabilities, and seniors. The health insurance coverage Medicaid provides ranges from prenatal and pediatric care, to preventive care aimed at stemming chronic diseases, to long term care services and supports. Federal financial support and flexibilities in program rules, along with new tools and options made available through the Affordable Care Act, have helped provide a platform for CMS and states to adopt a range of improvements and innovations in their Medicaid programs. Under the Affordable Care Act, Medicaid eligibility has been simplified and aligned across coverage programs. Thanks to these simplifications and the availability of Medicaid coverage to more low-income adults, millions more uninsured Americans are gaining coverage.

Because Medicaid is jointly funded by states and the Federal Government and is administered by states within Federal guidelines, both the Federal Government and states have key roles as stewards of the program, and CMS and states work together closely to carry out these responsibilities. Under the Medicaid Federal-state partnership, the Federal Government sets forth a policy framework for the program and states have significant flexibility to choose options that enable them to deliver high quality, cost-efficient care for their residents. CMS is committed to working with states and other partners to advance efforts that promote health, improve the quality of care, and lower health care costs.

This month we mark the 50th anniversary of the Medicaid program. For five decades, Medicaid has helped facilitate access to needed health services and provided financial security through protection from high out-of-pocket costs for millions of low-income Americans. Medicaid has played a vital role in providing comprehensive care for children that helps support their growth, school readiness, and development into healthy adults. Medicaid has also supported working families whose employers do not offer affordable health insurance, and fostered better health for pregnant women and positive birth outcomes for their babies by facilitating access to critical prenatal services. It has helped address the frequently complex health needs of people with disabilities, and supported them in living independently. And it has covered long-term care services and supports for millions of America's seniors and works in concert with Medicare to meet critical health needs. Over time, Medicaid has also risen to new challenges, providing care for people with HIV and AIDS, meeting the screening and treatment needs of people with breast and cervical cancer, and contributing to financial stability for low-income families by helping them maintain coverage during economic downturns.

Medicaid plays a fundamental role in assuring that low-income people have access to a high level of care. According to survey research released by the Commonwealth Fund last month, 95 percent of adults who had continuous Medicaid coverage in 2014 had a regular source of care, and the percentage of people who rated the quality of the care they received in the past 12 months as excellent or very good was comparable to that of people enrolled in private coverage. Adults enrolled in Medicaid also reported getting key preventive services like blood pressure checks at higher rates than did individuals who were uninsured. And Medicaid beneficiaries were less likely to have had problems paying medical bills than did individuals who had private coverage or who were uninsured. They were also less likely than those who were uninsured to skip getting medical care or to let a prescription go unfilled due to cost.[1]

Recent research that examined the long-term impact of Medicaid on the population it serves demonstrates that it is a sound investment for the Nation. Earlier this year, researchers at the National Bureau of Economic Research reported the results of longitudinal research that

---

[1] http://www.commonwealthfund.org/publications/issue-briefs/2015/jun/does-medicaid-make-a-difference

examined children enrolled in Medicaid and the Children's Health Insurance Program (CHIP) over time. They found that being enrolled in Medicaid and CHIP confers substantial benefits on individuals, and the country as a whole, when they reach adulthood. Specifically, the researchers found that individuals who were eligible for Medicaid and CHIP as children had higher cumulative wages as adults than their peers. The researchers estimated that the Federal Government recoups 56 cents of each dollar spent on childhood Medicaid by the time those children reach age 60.[2]

As we approach Medicaid's 50th anniversary, CMS is building on Medicaid's past successes and enhancing the program. Today I would like to highlight some of the key areas in which CMS is working with states to strengthen the program's ability to serve its beneficiaries:

- modernizing the eligibility and enrollment process for Medicaid and CHIP to support a strong consumer experience;
- expanding Medicaid eligibility to decrease the number of uninsured Americans and lower the costs of uncompensated care;
- strengthening payment and delivery systems reform to encourage coordinated, high quality, patient-centered care;
- continuing to advance the ability of seniors and people with disabilities to receive home and community-based care;
- updating the Medicaid managed care rules to promote quality, transparency, and access to care and to align with the rules of other payers;
- enhancing data systems to more accurately measure health care quality and strengthen program integrity and Medicaid financial management; and
- strengthening program integrity efforts to better combat and prevent fraud, waste, and abuse.

Modernizing Medicaid and CHIP Eligibility and Enrollment Processes
In our implementation of the Affordable Care Act, CMS has substantially simplified and modernized Medicaid and CHIP rules and processes for most people who apply for Medicaid and CHIP, creating an enrollment process that helps eligible consumers enroll in Medicaid and

---

[2] http://www.nber.org/papers/w20835

CHIP and access their coverage more quickly and smoothly. These rules are designed to align and coordinate with policies and procedures established for people who enroll in qualified health plans through the Marketplace. Before these changes, consumers would often encounter a paper-dependent process that was unnecessarily complex and time intensive, sometimes involving long waits for a decision on a family's eligibility that posed logistical challenges for working families and could delay access to needed care.

Now, consumers can use a single, streamlined application to apply for Medicaid, CHIP, and qualified health plans through the Marketplace. Consumers can apply online, over the phone, or by mail, and can get help from application assistors in their communities, or via call centers that help people apply for coverage. CMS and states have established an electronic approach to verifying financial and non-financial information needed to determine Medicaid, CHIP, and Marketplace eligibility. States now rely on available electronic data sources to confirm data included on the application, facilitating faster eligibility decisions and promoting program integrity. In addition, simplified renewal processes help ensure that people retain Medicaid and CHIP coverage for as long as they are eligible, and that beneficiaries who remain eligible get needed services like prescription medications.

Modernized state eligibility and enrollment systems underpin many of these simplifications by enabling automated eligibility verification, offering online applications and streamlining the consumer experience. To help states invest in these systems, CMS made available 90-percent matching funds through December 31, 2015, for eligibility system design and development, and the enhanced 75-percent matching rate indefinitely for maintenance and operations of such systems provided that these systems met certain standards and conditions that were designed to support a simple, streamlined enrollment process. In April, in a Notice of Proposed Rulemaking, CMS proposed ongoing access to the 90-percent and 75-percent matching authority for eligibility and enrollment systems to provide states with additional time to complete their full systems modernization, retire outdated "legacy" systems, and promote a dynamic, integrated, enterprise approach to Medicaid information technology systems. Refinements were made to the standards and conditions to ensure optimal systems development and efficient use of state and Federal funding.

As a result of these simplifications and systems improvements, states are making substantial progress processing Medicaid and CHIP applications more efficiently, often in real or near real-time. For example, in Washington, 92 percent of applications are processed in under 24 hours; in New York, 80 percent of applications are processed in one session; and in Rhode Island, 66 percent of applications are processed without manual intervention or the requirement of additional information.

Expanding Medicaid Eligibility

As a result of the Affordable Care Act, states have the opportunity to expand Medicaid eligibility to individuals ages 19-64 years of age with incomes up to 133 percent of the Federal poverty level (FPL). For the first time, states can provide Medicaid coverage for low-income adults without dependent children without the need for a demonstration waiver. The Affordable Care Act provides full Federal funding to cover newly eligible adults in states that expand Medicaid up to 133 percent FPL through Calendar Year 2016, and covers no less than 90 percent of costs thereafter. This increased Federal support has enabled 28 states and the District of Columbia to expand Medicaid coverage to more low-income adults. Most recently, in January, Indiana expanded its efforts to bring much needed access to health care coverage to uninsured low-income residents. Primarily as a result of the expansion of coverage to low-income adults and the eligibility and enrollment simplifications CMS and states have made, 12.3 million people have gained Medicaid or CHIP coverage since the beginning of the Affordable Care Act's first open enrollment period.[3]

States that have expanded their Medicaid programs are documenting significant reductions in uncompensated care and the uninsured rate. Hospitals provided over $50 billion in uncompensated care in 2013; in 2014, there was a $7.4 billion reduction in uncompensated care costs, and with 68 percent of the reduction coming from states expanding Medicaid.[4] And of the 11 states with the greatest reductions in uninsured rates in 2015, 10 had expanded Medicaid

---

[3] http://www.medicaid.gov/medicaid-chip-program-information/program-information/downloads/april-2015-enrollment-report.pdf
[4] http://aspe.hhs.gov/health/reports/2015/medicaidexpansion/ib_uncompensatedcare.pdf

eligibility.[5] This coverage is translating into tangible improvements in population health. Nearly one-third of the cases of diabetes in the United States have not been diagnosed; however, in states that expanded Medicaid, the number of beneficiaries with newly identified diabetes rose by 23 percent, compared to 0.4 percent in states that did not expand Medicaid, in the first six months of 2014.[6]

CMS is committed to working with states to expand Medicaid in ways that work for them, while protecting the integrity of the program and those it serves. For example, in Iowa and Arkansas, under section 1115(a) demonstrations, some new Medicaid enrollees receive their coverage from Qualified Health Plans offered in the individual market through the Marketplace. Michigan's Health and Wellness Plan promotes healthy behaviors through education and engagement of beneficiaries and providers. Iowa's demonstration includes a Healthy Behaviors program under which a beneficiary is eligible to reduce his/her premium payment amount by engaging in health improvement activities.

Accelerating States' Efforts on Medicaid Delivery System Reform

States and CMS share a strong interest in achieving better health and better care at lower cost. Medicaid plays a major role in the health care delivery system, and funds 16 percent of the Nation's health care services.[7] The expansion of Medicaid to new populations presents both states and CMS with additional opportunities to pursue delivery system reforms that improve the Medicaid patient experience while helping to drive innovation across the health care system. CMS is engaged in a variety of initiatives to work with states, providers, and other stakeholders to help spur innovation. CMS has collaborated with states in key areas to improve the quality of care and reform payment and delivery systems, has worked with innovator states to advance specific reforms, has provided states with tools and guidance developed to meet the needs of Medicaid beneficiaries, and is working to measure and improve quality across states, in coordination with similar efforts underway in Medicare and in the private market.

---

[5] http://www.gallup.com/poll/181664/arkansas-kentucky-improvement-uninsured-rates.aspx
[6] http://care.diabetesjournals.org/content/38/5/833.long
[7] http://kff.org/health-reform/issue-brief/medicaid-moving-forward/

Earlier this year, Department of Health and Human Services (HHS) Secretary Burwell announced measurable goals and a timeline to move the Medicare program, and the health care system at large, toward paying providers based on the quality, rather than the quantity of care they provide. This initiative will ultimately create a payment environment that appropriately promotes and rewards better care management for persons with chronic illness. CMS is dedicated to working with states to advance delivery system reforms that support these goals throughout the Medicaid and CHIP programs.

Strong Start

The Strong Start for Mothers and Newborns initiative includes two strategies to reduce premature births: first, working with hospitals to reduce the number of early elective deliveries across all payers; and second, testing models of enhanced prenatal care to reduce preterm births among women covered by Medicaid or CHIP.

The first strategy is a public-private partnership and awareness campaign to reduce the rate of non-medically indicated early elective deliveries prior to 39 weeks. Working together with Partnership for Patients, HHS sponsored public-private efforts to improve the safety, reliability, and cost of hospital care. The Partnership for Patients is an initiative that works with providers to identify potential hospital safety solutions and test models for improving care transitions from the hospital to other settings, and for reducing readmissions for high-risk Medicare beneficiaries. CMS collaborated with Hospital Engagement Networks, a group of providers that work at the regional, state, national, or hospital system level to help identify solutions already working and disseminate them to other hospitals and providers, across the country to identify and spread best practices to reduce potentially unnecessary early elective deliveries, which contributed to a 70.4-percent reduction in early elective deliveries between 2010 and 2013 among participating hospitals. For example, the Ohio Perinatal Quality Collaborative used a range of interventions to shift almost 21,000 births from between 36-38 weeks' gestation to 39 weeks gestation between September 2008 and October 2011. This shift reduced NICU admissions by three percent (approximately 621 admissions), which alone resulted in an estimated $24.8 million in savings for the three year period. Almost half of these births were to mothers enrolled in Medicaid.

The second Strong Start strategy is a four-year initiative to test new approaches to prenatal care and evaluate enhanced prenatal care interventions for women enrolled in Medicaid or CHIP who are at risk for having a preterm birth. The goal of the initiative is to determine if these approaches to care can reduce the rate of preterm births, improve the health outcomes of pregnant women and newborns, and decrease the anticipated total cost of medical care during pregnancy, delivery and over the first year of life. The initiative is currently supporting service delivery through 27 awardees and 213 provider sites, across 30 states, the District of Columbia, and Puerto Rico. While more thorough analysis must be completed, preliminary findings after year one of the program suggest that the enhanced prenatal care models may have a positive effect on some birth outcomes — specifically, increased rates of breastfeeding, decreased rates of cesarean section delivery, and decreased rates of preterm birth in comparison to national averages.

Health Homes

The Affordable Care Act created an optional Medicaid State Plan benefit that allows states to establish Health Homes in order to better coordinate care for people with Medicaid who have chronic conditions. Health Home providers operate under a "whole person" philosophy to integrate and coordinate all primary, acute, and behavioral health care, and long-term care services and supports, and to measure quality of care. Through this program, states receive a 90-percent enhanced Federal Medical Assistance Percentage (FMAP) for health home services for the first eight quarters and receive their regular match rate thereafter.

To date, CMS has approved Health Home State Plan Amendments in 19 states, the first of which was Missouri. Missouri's Medicaid program, in conjunction with its Department of Mental Health, successfully launched two Health Home initiatives: one designed to improve care for Medicaid beneficiaries with physical health conditions and one for beneficiaries with behavioral health conditions. Under these initiatives, participating Health Home providers delivered patient-centered culturally sensitive care, enhanced care management and care coordination across health care settings, and improved access to individual and family supports, including referral to community, social support, and recovery services. Missouri's Health Home programs reported reductions in-hospital admissions per 1000 of 12.8 percent and 5.9 percent, respectively, while emergency-room usage per 1000 also declined by 8.2 percent and 9.7 percent in each program. The state is also reporting an improvement in several key clinical indicators, including hemoglobin A1C levels in participants with diabetes mellitus, as well as LDL cholesterol levels and systolic and diastolic blood pressures in participants with heart disease.

Innovative State Delivery System Models

Many State Medicaid agencies have started using a variety of approaches to improve and modernize their delivery and payment systems. For example, in 2012, Oregon launched a new managed care model, creating Coordinated Care Organizations (CCOs) that are risk-bearing, locally-governed provider networks that deliver community-driven coordinated care to Medicaid beneficiaries. These entities provide all Medicaid enrollees with physical, behavioral, and dental health services. The CCOs are paid via a global Medicaid budget that grows at a fixed rate, while allowing for some flexibility in the services that a plan provides. Oregon is held to quality and spending metrics to ensure that quality continues to improve as the state and CCOs control costs. The CCOs are held accountable for performance-based metrics and quality standards that align with industry standards, new systems of governance, and payment incentives that reward improved health outcomes. CMS has also worked with states to advance integrated care models like patient centered medical homes and accountable care organizations.

Delivery System Reform Incentive Program

CMS works with interested states to pursue state-initiated and developed delivery system reform initiatives. Through Delivery System Reform Incentive Payment (DSRIP) programs, authorized through section 1115(a) demonstrations, states support hospitals and other providers in enhancing how they provide Medicaid services. The first DSRIP initiatives were approved in 2010, and the most recent initiative will begin this year. The lessons learned over this period of time have helped CMS to refine the DSRIP initiatives and focus them on sustainable, beneficiary-focused changes to how providers are organized and how care is paid for under the Medicaid program. Currently, eight states have section 1115(a) demonstrations with DSRIP programs.

These initiatives are continuing to evolve, with the most recently approved DSRIP program providing funding for a broader set of providers, more specific evaluation metrics, and requirements to meet statewide goals. CMS will continue to work with these states to design and evaluate both short- and long-term outcomes of these initiatives and the impacts they are having on care delivery, the costs of services, and the overall health of Medicaid beneficiaries.

Medicaid Innovation Accelerator Program

To spur innovation between CMS and the states, CMS created the Medicaid Innovation Accelerator Program (IAP) with the goal of improving health and health care for Medicaid beneficiaries by supporting states' ongoing payment and service delivery-reform efforts. The IAP is consistent with recommendations made by the National Governors Association Health Care Sustainability Task Force, which focused on system transformation and state innovations that rely on the redesign of health care delivery and payment systems. Through the IAP, states can receive targeted program support designed around their ongoing delivery and payment system-innovation efforts.

CMS selected four areas as IAP's program priorities in consultation with states and stakeholders: (1) substance use disorders; (2) Medicaid beneficiaries with high needs and high costs; (3) community integration to support long-term services and supports; and (4) physical and mental health integration. CMS has been working intensively with seven states over the past five months on the first priority area to develop and implement substance use disorder service delivery reform activities. Additionally, CMS announced the details of the second IAP program priority area, improving care for Medicaid beneficiaries with complex needs and high costs, at the end of June 2015 via a national webinar. The final two program priority areas, community integration to support long- term services and supports and physical and mental health integration, have target launch timeframes of fall and winter of 2015, respectively. CMS also is working with some states to support data integration across Medicare and Medicaid to provide integrated care for Medicare-Medicaid enrollees.

All states can be laboratories for health care reform. As noted above, 19 states have initiated comprehensive health homes for people with multiple chronic conditions. Several states have developed shared savings payment models through State Innovation Models. Twelve states are testing new delivery and payment models for people who are dually eligible for Medicaid and Medicare through the Financial Alignment Initiative. While payment and service delivery innovation is well underway in states, there are common challenges to all Medicaid delivery reforms, particularly in technical areas such as data analytics, payment modeling and financial simulations, quality measurement, and rapid cycle learning. IAP will help strengthen all of our efforts on delivery reform and move Medicaid payment and delivery to the next level by addressing these shared issues.

State Innovation Models

The CMS Innovation Center created the State Innovation Models (SIM) initiative for states that are prepared for or committed to planning, designing, testing, and supporting evaluation of new payment and service delivery models in the context of larger health system transformation. The SIM is providing financial and technical support to states for the development and testing of state-led, multi-payer health care payment and service delivery models that will improve health system performance, increase quality of care, and decrease costs for Medicare, Medicaid and CHIP beneficiaries.

In Round One of the SIM Initiative, 25 states were awarded funds to design or test innovative health care payment and service delivery models in the form of Model Design, Model Pre-Test, and Model Test awards. In Round Two,[8] the SIM Initiative is providing funds to 28 states, three territories, and the District of Columbia. This includes both Model Design awardees, states that are designing plans and strategies for statewide innovation, and Model Test awardees, states that are testing and implementing comprehensive statewide health transformation plans. Including the Round Two awardees, over half of states, representing 61 percent of the U.S. population, will be working to support comprehensive state-based innovation in health system transformation. Many of the states participating in SIM are developing new approaches to delivering care to Medicaid and CHIP beneficiaries. For example, in Maine, the SIM grant from CMS has supported the state to design a vision for a robust multi-payer model, including components such as health homes and shared savings.

---

[8] For more information: http://innovation.cms.gov/initiatives/State-Innovations-Round-Two/index.html

Financial Alignment Initiative

Today there are over 10 million Americans enrolled in both the Medicare and Medicaid programs, commonly known as "dual eligible" beneficiaries. The Medicare-Medicaid Financial Alignment Initiative is designed to better align the financial incentives of the two programs to provide these dual eligible beneficiaries with improved health outcomes and a better care experience.

The Financial Alignment Initiative created two model types: capitated and managed fee-for-service. In the capitated model, a state, CMS, and a health plan enter into a three-way contract, and the plan receives a prospective blended payment to provide comprehensive, coordinated care. In the managed fee-for-service model, a state and CMS enter into an agreement by which the state is eligible to benefit from a portion of savings from initiatives designed to improve quality and reduce costs for both Medicare and Medicaid. Implementation of each demonstration is a collaborative effort between CMS and the state, and CMS has made several resources available to assist states with implementation activities. To date, new demonstrations are underway in 12 states, with approximately 400,000 dually-eligible beneficiaries participating in the financial-alignment models.

Moving Towards Home and Community-Based Care

CMS continues to look for ways to enable Medicaid beneficiaries with disabilities to receive home and community-based care, instead of relying on institutional care. The commitment to deliver care in ways that improve both efficiency and beneficiary outcomes extends beyond the delivery of acute and outpatient care to the delivery of long term care services as well. The passage of the Affordable Care Act provides new and expanded opportunities to serve more individuals in home and community-based settings.

The core mechanism that states have used to promote access to community-based services and supports for Medicaid beneficiaries is through Home and Community-Based Services (HCBS) waivers. Today, 47 states and Washington, D.C. operate at least one 1915(c) HCBS waiver. The Affordable Care Act also created new options under state plan authority for states to provide home and community-based care. For example, the Affordable Care Act authorized Community First Choice under section 1915(k), a state plan benefit that offers community-based attendant supports and services to individuals who meet institutional levels of care. Five states have approved Community First Choice state plan amendments and CMS is also working intensively with several additional states on proposals that are under review.

As states continue to reduce their reliance on institutional care, develop community-based long-term care opportunities, and transition individuals living in institutions to community living, almost all of them have worked with CMS as part of our Money Follows the Person Rebalancing Demonstration Grant Program. Today, 43 states and Washington, D.C. participate in Money Follows the Person and receive enhanced Federal matching funds to serve individuals who move from institutional care to community integrated long-term care settings. In addition to Money Follows the Person, 18 states currently participate in the Balancing Incentive Program, also created by the Affordable Care Act, which provides enhanced Federal match to states that make structural reforms to increase institutional diversion and access to non-institutional long-term care services. According to the forthcoming Long-Term Services and Supports (LTSS) Expenditure Report to be released by CMS, 2013 data show that Medicaid spending on such services has tipped in favor of the community, with51 percent spent on community-based services versus 49 percent being spent on institutional services. Ten years ago, community-based spending made up just 33 percent of total long-term care spending.

Medicaid has also helped ensure that individuals are the focal point of the HCBS care planning process and that they have choice of and control over HCBS services. HCBS programs have a person-centered planning requirement – a process directed by the individual with long-term care service and support needs which may include a representative chosen by the individual, and/or who is authorized to make personal or health decisions for the person, family members, legal guardians, friends, caregivers, and others the person or his/her representative wishes to include. HCBS programs also include the ability for an individual to "self-direct" their services. Participant or self-directed service options in long-term care financing programs provide individuals and their representatives the opportunity to hire, manage, and fire their direct-service workers. Funds may also be used to purchase other goods and services, such as assistive technology, home modifications, personal care supplies, and transportation, within Federal and state guidelines. At least 38 states have self-direction programs in place for HCBS and about one quarter of all Medicaid beneficiaries receiving HCBS are self-directing some of their services, according to state-reported data in 2014.

As we move to more home and community-based services, acknowledging that the majority of Medicaid spending is in the area of long-term care services and supports, CMS is engaged in making sure that the delivery of these services is supported by robust data. As such, we are engaged in testing an experience of care survey and a set of functional assessment elements, demonstrating the use of personal health records and creating a standard electronic long-term services and support plan. This work will provide national metrics and valuable feedback on how health information technology can be implemented in this component of the Medicaid program.

Updating Managed Care

As the health care delivery system moves towards more integrated care and away from fee-for-service, states are increasingly moving to the use of managed care in serving Medicaid beneficiaries. Approximately 58 percent of Medicaid beneficiaries are enrolled in capitated, risk-based managed care for part or all of their services. Managed care is serving new populations, including seniors and people with disabilities who need long-term services and supports, and individuals newly eligible for Medicaid. Recognizing these changes, in May CMS issued a proposed rule to modernize Medicaid and CHIP managed care regulations to update the programs' rules and strengthen the delivery of quality care for beneficiaries. This proposed rule is the first major update to Medicaid and CHIP managed care regulations in more than a decade and a major part of CMS' efforts to strengthen delivery systems that serve Medicaid and CHIP beneficiaries.

The proposed rule incorporates several core principles to update the regulations, specifically aligning with Medicare Advantage and private coverage plans, supporting state delivery system reform, promoting the quality of care, strengthening program and fiscal integrity, incorporating best practices for managed long-term services and supports programs, and enhancing the beneficiary experience. Under the proposed rule, Medicaid managed care policies would be aligned to a much greater extent with those of Medicare Advantage and the private market, which would improve operational efficiencies for states and health plans, as well as improve the experience of care for individuals who transition between health care coverage options.

The proposed rule promotes state delivery system reform through encouraging initiatives within managed care programs that strive to improve health care outcomes and beneficiary experience while controlling costs. The proposed rule acknowledges the greater demand of mental health and substance abuse disorder services by clarifying that states are permitted to make a monthly capitation payment to a managed care plan for an enrollee that has a short term stay (no more than 15 days) in an institution for mental disease. The proposed rule would require a quality strategy for a state's entire Medicaid program and also establish a Medicaid managed care quality rating system that would include performance information on all health plans and align with the existing rating systems in Medicare Advantage and the Marketplace. By clarifying actuarial soundness requirements, CMS intends to strengthen fiscal and programmatic integrity of Medicaid managed care programs and rate setting. CMS also intends to implement best practices identified in existing managed long-term services and supports programs. The proposed rule would improve the beneficiary experience by making additional information and support systems available to individuals as they enroll in managed care. The proposed rule also supports beneficiaries by strengthening requirements on managed care plans to ensure that covered services are available and that individuals get high-quality, coordinated care through efforts such as strengthening network adequacy. In order to ensure CHIP beneficiaries the same quality and access in managed care programs, where appropriate, CHIP managed care regulations would be largely aligned with the proposed revisions to the Medicaid managed care rules.

Building Enhanced Data Systems

Improving and enhancing Medicaid data systems is an important part of CMS efforts to modernize the program. Better data systems can help both CMS and states measure health care quality and improve program integrity and Medicaid financial management. CMS has encouraged and supported states in their efforts to modernize and improve state Medicaid Management Information Systems, which will produce greater efficiencies and strengthen program integrity. CMS also developed the Transformed Medicaid Statistical Information System (T-MSIS). T-MSIS will facilitate state submission of timely claims data to HHS, expand the MSIS dataset, and allow CMS to review the completeness and quality of State MSIS submittals. CMS will explore using this data for the Medicaid improper payment measurement, evaluating section 1115 waivers and models being tested by the CMS Innovation Center, and to satisfy other HHS requirements. Through the use of T-MSIS, CMS will not only acquire higher quality data, but will also reduce state data requests. States will move from MSIS to T-MSIS on a rolling basis with the goal of having all states submitting data in the T-MSIS file format by the end of 2015.

Strengthening Program Integrity

CMS is committed to sound financial management of the Medicaid program and works to ensure that we are good stewards of taxpayer dollars. States and the Federal Government share mutual obligations and accountability for the integrity of the Medicaid program and the development, application, and improvement of program safeguards necessary to ensure proper and appropriate use of both Federal and State dollars. This Federal-State partnership is central to the success of the Medicaid program, and it depends on clear lines of responsibility and shared expectations. Through provisions included in the Affordable Care Act and through CMS regulations, we are enhancing program integrity by strengthening provider and beneficiary eligibility safeguards, as well as by maintaining strong oversight partnerships and data exchanges with states. For example, the Affordable Care Act required CMS to implement risk-based screening of providers and suppliers who want to participate in Medicare, Medicaid, and CHIP.

HHS has implemented a Comprehensive Medicaid Integrity Plan (CMIP), which provides a strategy for CMS to improve Medicaid program integrity for the FY 2014-2018 period.[9] The execution of the strategies in CMIP will improve the ability of state Medicaid agencies and CMS to leverage program data to detect and prevent improper payments, which will strengthen the ability of state Medicaid agencies to safeguard state and Federal Medicaid dollars from diversion into fraud, waste, and abuse. In addition, CMS is working to streamline its assessments of state Medicaid program integrity activities. CMS began conducting comprehensive state program

---

[9] http://www.cms.gov/Regulations-and-Guidance/Legislation/DeficitReductionAct/Downloads/cmip2014.pdf

integrity reviews in 2007 on a triennial basis. These reviews play a critical role in how CMS provides assistance to states in their efforts to combat provider fraud and abuse.

Confronting Challenges and Moving Forward

Throughout its 50-year history, Medicaid has served as an adaptable program, adjusting to national and state-specific needs and meeting the health care needs of children, adults, pregnant women, seniors, and people with disabilities. For these low-income Americans, Medicaid has provided health insurance coverage that is affordable, accessible, and has served as the Nation's major source of long-term care coverage. CMS will continue to work closely with states and other stakeholders to continue to strengthen the Medicaid program in key areas such as modernizing the enrollment process; strengthening delivery systems and managed care; increasing our collection and use of data to make policy and program-management decisions; and enabling individuals with disabilities to live in their homes and communities.

I appreciate the Subcommittee's ongoing interest in the Medicaid program, and look forward to working with you to strengthen and improve Medicaid for the people the program serves.

Mr. PITTS. The Chair thanks the gentlelady. I now recognize Ms. Yocom, 5 minutes for your opening statement.

STATEMENT OF CAROLYN L. YOCOM

Ms. YOCOM. Chairman Pitts, Ranking Member Green, and members of the subcommittee, I am pleased to be here today with my colleague, Katherine Iritani, to discuss the key issues that are facing the Medicaid program. Today Medicaid is undergoing a period of transformative change as enrollment grows following the passage of the Patient Protection and Affordable Care Act. Under this Act, more than half of the States have elected to expand their Medicaid programs and cover low-income adults who were not previously eligible for the program.

At the heart of Medicaid is a Federal/State partnership. Both the Federal Government and the States play important roles in ensuring that Medicaid is fiscally responsible and sustainable over time, and effective in meeting the needs of its population that it serves. We designated Medicaid as a high-risk program in 2003, and our statement highlights some of the significant oversight challenges that, based on our work, exist today.

Our statement highlights four key issues: First, access to care; second, transparency and oversight; third, program integrity; and fourth, Federal financing. Congress and HHS have taken some positive steps related to these four key issues, and continued attention is critical to ensure that the Medicaid program is effective for the enrollees who rely on it, and also accountable to the taxpayers who pay for it. Accordingly, our work recommends additional steps to bolster efforts in each of these areas.

First, maintaining and improving access to care is critical to ensuring that Medicaid operates effectively. Our analysis of national survey data suggests that access to care in Medicaid is generally comparable to that of individuals with private insurance. However, our work also shows that Medicaid enrollees can face particular challenges accessing certain types of care, such as mental health and dental care.

Second, increased transparency and improved oversight can help improve the Medicaid program. For example, CMS lacks complete and reliable data about the sources of funds that States use to finance the non-Federal share of Medicaid, and it also lacks complete data on payments to providers, which hinders oversight. Gaps in HHS' criteria, process, and policy for improving State spending on demonstration projects also raises added questions about tens of billions of dollars in Federal spending.

Third, improving program integrity can help ensure the most appropriate use of Medicaid funds. Improper payments are a significant cost to Medicaid, totaling an estimated 17.5 billion in fiscal year 2014. Our work suggests that an effective Federal/State partnership is a key factor in improper payments and combating them, not only to oversee spending in both fee-for-service and managed care, but also to set appropriate payment rates for managed care organizations, and ensure that only eligible individuals and providers participate in Medicaid.

Fourth, since its inception, efforts to finance the Medicaid program have been in odds with the cyclical nature of its design and operation, particularly during national economic downturns. We suggested that Congress consider enacting a Federal funding formula that would provide automatic, targeted, and timely assistance to States during national economic downturns. We have also described revisions to the current Federal funding formula that could more equitably allocate Medicaid funds to States by better accounting for each State's ability to finance the program.

In conclusion, continued focus on these challenges is critical to ensuring that continued access to care for the tens of millions of Americans who are in the Medicaid program. It is also critical to ensuring the sustainability. Chairman Pitts, Ranking Member Green, and members of the subcommittee, this concludes our prepared statement. We would be pleased to respond to any questions you might have.

[The prepared statement of Ms. Yocom follows:]

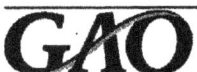

United States Government Accountability Office

Testimony

Before the Subcommittee on Health, Committee on Energy and Commerce, House of Representatives

For Release on Delivery
Expected at 10:15 a.m. ET
Wednesday, July 8, 2015

MEDICAID

Overview of Key Issues Facing the Program

Statement of Katherine M. Iritani
Director, Health Care

Carolyn L. Yocom
Director, Health Care

July 8, 2015

MEDICAID

Overview of Key Issues Facing the Program

What GAO Found

GAO identified four key issues facing the Medicaid program: access to care; transparency and oversight; program integrity; and federal financing.

- **Access to care:** Medicaid enrollees report access to care that is generally comparable to privately insured individuals, but may have greater difficulty accessing specialty care (like mental health care) and dental care. GAO has recommended actions such as improving data on enrollees' access to care. CMS has issued guidance to states about reporting referrals for services, but has no plans to require states to report whether certain enrollees receive services for which they are referred, as GAO recommended.

- **Transparency and oversight:** The lack of reliable CMS data on states' financing of the non-federal share of Medicaid and program payments to providers hinders federal oversight, and GAO has recommended steps to improve data and oversight. Also, improvements are needed in the Department of Health and Human Services' (HHS) criteria, policy, and process for approving states' spending on demonstrations—state projects that may test new ways to deliver or pay for care, which have grown to account for close to one-third of federal Medicaid spending in 2014. HHS has approved demonstration spending limits that were not budget neutral to the federal government, as required by HHS policy. GAO estimated that spending limits were tens of billions of dollars higher than what spending would have been if states' existing Medicaid programs had continued. GAO has suggested that Congress consider requiring HHS to make improvements in these areas, such as by better ensuring that valid methods are used to demonstrate budget neutrality.

- **Program integrity:** The program's size and diversity make it vulnerable to improper payments, which totaled an estimated $17.5 billion in fiscal year 2014, according to HHS. Key to ensuring the most appropriate use of funds are (1) identifying and preventing improper payments in fee-for-service and managed care, (2) setting appropriate payment rates for managed care organizations, and (3) ensuring only eligible individuals and providers participate in Medicaid. GAO has recommended steps to improve program integrity, such as by improving Medicaid managed care oversight. CMS has taken some steps, but the lack of a comprehensive program integrity strategy for managed care leaves a growing portion of Medicaid funds at risk. GAO believes that further actions, such as requiring states to conduct audits of payments to and by managed care organizations, are crucial.

- **Federal financing:** Automatic temporary increases in federal assistance during economic downturns and more equitable allocations of federal Medicaid funds to states (by better accounting for states' ability to fund Medicaid) could better align federal funding with states' needs, offering states greater fiscal stability. GAO has suggested that Congress could consider enacting a funding formula that provides automatic, targeted, and timely assistance in response to national economic downturns. GAO has also described revisions to the current funding formula that could better align federal funding with each state's resources, demand for services, and costs.

Why GAO Did This Study

The Medicaid program marks its 50th anniversary on July 30, 2015. The joint federal-state program has grown to be one of the largest sources of health care coverage and financing for a diverse low-income and medically needy population. Medicaid is a significant component of federal and state budgets, with estimated outlays of $508 billion in fiscal year 2014, of which $304 billion was financed by the federal government and $204 billion by the states. The program is a federal-state partnership, and both the federal government and the states play important roles in ensuring that Medicaid is fiscally sustainable over time and effective in meeting the needs of the populations it serves. GAO considers Medicaid a high-risk program due to its size, growth, diversity, and gaps in oversight identified by GAO's work.

GAO has a large body of work on challenges facing Medicaid, and on gaps in federal oversight. This testimony addresses key issues that face the Medicaid program based on this work. It is based on GAO reports on Medicaid issued from January 2005 through June 2015, and information from the Centers for Medicare & Medicaid Services (CMS), the HHS agency that oversees Medicaid, about the status of prior GAO recommendations.

GAO has made over 80 recommendations regarding Medicaid. HHS has taken action in response to some of GAO's prior recommendations, but did not agree with others. GAO continues to believe that its recommendations have merit and should be implemented.

View GAO-15-746T. For more information, contact Katherine M. Iritani at (202) 512-7114 or iritanik@gao.gov or Carolyn L. Yocom at (202) 512-7114 or yocomc@gao.gov.

Highlights of GAO-15-746T, a testimony before the Subcommittee on Health, Committee on Energy and Commerce, House of Representatives

United States Government Accountability Office

Chairman Pitts, Ranking Member Green, and Members of the
Subcommittee:

We are pleased to be here today to discuss key issues facing the
Medicaid program. The Medicaid program marks its 50th anniversary on
July 30, 2015. Over the past half-century, Medicaid has grown to be one
of the largest sources of health care coverage and financing for a diverse
low-income and medically needy population. Medicaid is a significant
component of federal and state budgets, with estimated outlays of
$508 billion in fiscal year 2014, of which $304 billion was financed by
the federal government and $204 billion by the states.[1] Operating as an
important health care safety net, Medicaid covered about 72 million
individuals—roughly one-fifth of the U.S. population—during fiscal year
2013.[2] Medicaid is undergoing a period of transformative change, as
enrollment is growing under the Patient Protection and Affordable Care
Act (PPACA). In particular, PPACA permits states to expand their
Medicaid programs by covering certain low-income adults not historically
eligible for Medicaid coverage, and more than half of the states have
done so.

Medicaid is designed as a federal-state partnership, and both the federal
government and the states play important roles in ensuring that Medicaid
is fiscally sustainable over time and effective in meeting the needs of the
vulnerable populations it serves. Medicaid is financed jointly by the
federal government and states, administered at the state level, and
overseen at the federal level by the Centers for Medicare & Medicaid
Services (CMS), within the Department of Health and Human Services
(HHS). By design, Medicaid allows significant flexibility for states to
design and implement their programs. While state flexibility is a key
element of the program, federal oversight is important to help ensure that
funds are used appropriately and that enrollees can access quality care.
However, significant challenges for oversight exist, given the size, growth,

---

[1]Centers for Medicare & Medicaid Services, Office of the Actuary, *2013 Actuarial Report
on the Financial Outlook for Medicaid* (Washington, D.C.: 2014). As of June 30, 2015, the
Centers for Medicare & Medicaid Services had not published data on final fiscal year 2014
expenditures.

[2]This figure represents the total number of individuals ever enrolled in the program in
2013. There were about 58 million individuals enrolled in the program at any one point in
time. See Medicaid and CHIP Payment and Access Commission, *Report to the Congress
on Medicaid and CHIP* (Washington, D.C.: March 2014).

and diversity of Medicaid, which we designated as a high-risk program in 2003 due to these factors and gaps in oversight we identified.

Over the years, we have reported on a number of challenges facing Medicaid, and made numerous recommendations regarding gaps in federal oversight of the program.[3] Our statement today highlights key issues that face the Medicaid program, based on our work. To identify the key issues for this statement, we reviewed more than 70 reports on Medicaid that we issued from January 2005 through June 2015, including our most recent high risk update, which provides an overview of challenges facing Medicaid and areas needing improved federal oversight.[4] From January 2015 to May 2015, we also obtained and reviewed information from CMS about the status of our prior recommendations, as well as current CMS efforts related to Medicaid.[5] The issues we discuss are neither inclusive of all the issues facing Medicaid nor all the issues CMS faces in its oversight efforts. We conducted all of the work on which this statement is based in accordance with generally accepted government auditing standards. Those standards require that we plan and perform the audit to obtain sufficient, appropriate evidence to provide a reasonable basis for our findings and conclusions based on our audit objectives. We believe that the evidence obtained provides a reasonable basis for our findings and conclusions based on our audit objectives.

In summary, we found that the Medicaid program faces a range of key issues as it marks its 50th year. Attention to these key issues—access to care; transparency and oversight; program integrity; and federal financing—will be important to ensuring that the Medicaid program is both effective for the enrollees who rely on it and accountable to the taxpayers. Matters for congressional consideration and selected GAO recommendations that address these key issues are summarized in appendix I.

[3]See, for example, GAO, *High-Risk Series: An Update*, GAO-15-290 (Washington, D.C.: Feb. 11, 2015).

[4]See the list of related GAO products at the end of this statement for selected reports about Medicaid.

[5]See Appendix I for selected prior GAO recommendations regarding Medicaid. GAO has made over 80 recommendations regarding Medicaid.

Access to care. Maintaining and improving access to care is critical to ensuring that the program is effective for the individuals who rely on it. National survey data have suggested that access to medical care reported by Medicaid enrollees is generally comparable to that of individuals with private health insurance—with few (less than 4 percent) reporting difficulty obtaining necessary medical care in 2008 and 2009—but that Medicaid enrollees do face particular challenges in accessing certain types of care, such as obtaining specialty care (like mental health care) or dental care.[6] For example, our 2010 national survey of physicians found that specialty physicians were generally more willing to accept privately insured children as new patients than Medicaid-covered children, and that more physicians reported having difficulty referring Medicaid-covered children to specialty providers than reported having difficulty referring privately insured children.[7] CMS has taken steps to help ensure enrollees' access to care, and we have recommended additional steps that could bolster those efforts. For example, in April 2011 we recommended CMS take steps to improve its data from states to help assess Medicaid enrollees' access to care.[8] In particular, we recommended that CMS work with states to explore options for capturing information on children's receipt of services for which they were referred. The agency has issued guidance to states about how to report referrals for health care services, but has no plans to require states to report whether children receive services for which they are referred. We continue to believe this information is important for monitoring and ensuring children's access to care.

---

[6]See, for example, GAO, *Children's Health Insurance: Information on Coverage of Services, Costs to Consumers, and Access to Care in CHIP and Other Sources of Insurance*, GAO-14-40 (Washington, D.C.: Nov. 21, 2013); *Children's Mental Health: Concerns Remain about Appropriate Services for Children in Medicaid and Foster Care*, GAO-13-15 (Washington, D.C.: Dec. 10, 2012); and *Medicaid: States Made Multiple Program Changes, and Beneficiaries Generally Reported Access Comparable to Private Insurance*, GAO-13-55 (Washington, D.C.: Nov. 15, 2012).

[7]See GAO, *Medicaid and CHIP: Most Physicians Serve Covered Children but Have Difficulty Referring Them for Specialty Care*, GAO-11-624 (Washington, D.C.: June 30, 2011).

[8]See GAO, *Medicaid and CHIP: Reports for Monitoring Children's Health Care Services Need Improvement*, GAO-11-293R (Washington, D.C.: April 5, 2011).

Transparency and oversight. Efforts to ensure fiscal accountability through increased transparency and improved oversight can help ensure the appropriate use of Medicaid funds. States are responsible for financing the non-federal share of their programs, and can use state general funds as well as other sources, such as taxes on health care providers and transfers of funds from local governments. However, we have found CMS lacks complete and reliable data about the sources of funds states use to finance the non-federal share of Medicaid, including data needed to monitor states' reliance on providers and local governments to finance the non-federal share, which can shift costs to the federal government. CMS also lacks complete data on program payments to providers, which hinders oversight. Accordingly, our work has pointed to the need for better data on states' funding sources and state payments to providers, as well as improved policy and oversight.[9] In addition, we have highlighted the need for improvements in HHS's criteria, policy, and process for approving states' spending on demonstrations—state projects that may test new ways to deliver or pay for Medicaid benefits, which have grown over time to account for close to one-third of federal Medicaid spending in 2014.[10] Although HHS policy requires demonstrations to be budget-neutral to the federal government, HHS has approved demonstration spending limits that we estimate were billions of dollars higher than what federal spending would have been if the states' existing Medicaid programs had continued. We found that HHS has allowed states to use questionable methods and assumptions for their spending estimates, without providing adequate documentation to support them. We have also found that HHS has not issued explicit criteria explaining how it determines that demonstration spending furthers Medicaid objectives, and that HHS's approval documents are not always clear as to what, precisely, approved expenditures are for and how they will promote

---

[9]See, for example, GAO, *Medicaid: CMS Oversight of Provider Payments Is Hampered by Limited Data and Unclear Policy*, GAO-15-322 (Washington, D.C.: April 10, 2015); *Medicaid Financing: States' Increased Reliance on Funds from Health Care Providers and Local Governments Warrants Improved CMS Data Collection*, GAO-14-627 (Washington, D.C.: July 29, 2014); and *Medicaid: More Transparency of and Accountability for Supplemental Payments Are Needed*, GAO-13-48 (Washington, D.C.: Nov. 26, 2012).

[10]See, for example, GAO, *Medicaid Demonstrations: Approval Criteria and Documentation Need to Show How Spending Furthers Medicaid Objectives*, GAO-15-239 (Washington, D.C.: April 13, 2015); *Medicaid Demonstrations: HHS's Approval Process for Arkansas's Medicaid Expansion Waiver Raises Cost Concerns*, GAO-14-689R (Washington, D.C.: Aug. 8, 2014); and *Medicaid Demonstration Waivers: Approval Process Raises Cost Concerns and Lacks Transparency*, GAO-13-384 (Washington, D.C.: June 25, 2013).

37

these objectives.[11] As a result, the bases for HHS's decisions involving tens of billions of Medicaid dollars are not transparent.

Congress and HHS have taken important steps in recent years to improve transparency, oversight, and fiscal accountability, and we have recommended additional steps that would build on those efforts. For example, in July 2014, we recommended that CMS take steps to ensure that states report accurate and complete information on all sources of funds used to finance the nonfederal share of Medicaid, and offered suggestions for doing so. HHS disagreed, stating that its current efforts were adequate.[12] However, we continue to believe that improved data are needed to improve transparency and oversight. In addition, in April 2015, we recommended that CMS take steps to ensure that states report accurate and complete provider-specific payment data and develop a policy and process for reviewing payments to individual providers to determine whether they are economical and efficient, and HHS concurred with our recommendations.[13] In November 2012, we suggested that, because CMS said legislation was required for the agency to take particular steps to improve oversight of certain high-risk Medicaid payments, Congress consider requiring CMS to improve reporting of these payments and subject them to independent audit.[14] We also have made multiple recommendations aimed at improving HHS's demonstration approval process, such as by improving its review criteria and methods. In 2008, because HHS disagreed that our recommended changes were needed—maintaining that its process was sufficient—we suggested that Congress consider requiring the Secretary of HHS to take certain actions to improve the demonstration approval process, such as by better ensuring that valid methods are used to demonstrate budget neutrality, and documenting the basis for such approvals.[15] In April 2015, we recommended that HHS ensure that its demonstration approvals document the criteria used to assess whether demonstrations are likely to

---

[11]See GAO-15-239.

[12]See GAO-14-627.

[13]See GAO-15-322.

[14]See GAO-13-48.

[15]See GAO, *Medicaid Demonstration Waivers: Recent HHS Approvals Continue to Raise Cost and Oversight Concerns*, GAO-08-87 (Washington, D.C.: Jan. 31, 2008).

promote Medicaid objectives, and HHS concurred with this recommendation.[16]

Program integrity. Improving program integrity can help ensure the most appropriate use of Medicaid funds. The program's size and diversity make it particularly vulnerable to improper payments, including payments made for treatments or services that were not covered by the program, that were not medically necessary, or that were never provided. Improper payments are a significant cost to Medicaid—totaling an estimated $17.5 billion in fiscal year 2014, according to HHS. An effective federal-state partnership is key to ensuring the most appropriate use of funds by (1) identifying and preventing improper payments in both fee-for-service and managed care, (2) setting appropriate payment rates for managed care organizations, and (3) ensuring only eligible individuals and providers participate in Medicaid.[17] CMS has taken steps to improve program integrity, and we have recommended other steps that would bolster those efforts. In May 2014, for example, we recommended CMS take steps to improve oversight of growing Medicaid managed care expenditures.[18] CMS has taken some steps, but the lack of a comprehensive program integrity strategy for managed care leaves a growing portion of Medicaid funds at risk. We believe that further actions, in particular requiring states to conduct audits of payments to and by managed care organizations, and updating guidance on Medicaid managed care program integrity practices, are crucial to improving program integrity.

Federal financing. Medicaid's federal-state partnership could be improved through a revised federal financing approach that better addresses variations in states' financing needs. The federal government shares in the costs of state Medicaid payments using the Federal Medical

---

[16] See GAO-15-239.

[17] See, for example, GAO, *Medicaid: Additional Actions Needed to Help Improve Provider and Beneficiary Fraud Controls*, GAO-15-313 (Washington, D.C.: May 14, 2015); *Medicaid Information Technology: CMS Supports Use of Program Integrity Systems but Should Require States to Determine Effectiveness*, GAO-15-207 (Washington, D.C.: Jan. 30, 2015); *Medicaid: Additional Federal Action Needed to Further Improper Third-Party Liability Efforts*, GAO-15-208 (Washington, D.C.: Jan. 28, 2015); and *Medicaid Program Integrity: Increased Oversight Needed to Ensure Integrity of Growing Managed Care Expenditures*, GAO-14-341 (Washington, D.C.: May 19, 2014).

[18] See GAO-14-341.

Assistance Percentage (FMAP), which is determined annually by a statutory formula based in part on each state's per capita income. States with lower per capita incomes receive higher matching rates. Automatically providing increased federal financial assistance to states affected by national economic downturns, in a timely and targeted way—through temporary changes to the federal funding formula—could help provide assistance that is more responsive to states' particular economic conditions than past federal assistance when Congress acted to temporarily increase support to states by increasing the share of Medicaid expenditures paid by the federal government.[19] We suggested in November 2011 that Congress could consider enacting a federal funding formula that provides such automatic, targeted and timely assistance.[20] In addition, we have described revisions to the current federal funding formula that could more equitably allocate Medicaid funds to states by better accounting for their ability to fund Medicaid.[21] These improvements could better align federal funding with each state's resources, demand for services, and costs; better facilitate state budget planning; and provide states with greater fiscal stability during times of economic stress.

In conclusion, our previous work highlights the range of challenges facing the Medicaid program as it approaches its 50th anniversary. Addressing these challenges is critical to ensuring continued access to care for tens of millions of Americans and the fiscal sustainability of the program. In the coming weeks, we will issue a report that discusses these challenges—and recommendations we made in prior work to address them—in greater detail. The report will also describe the Medicaid program's ongoing transformation, as federal and state governments implement PPACA changes, prepare for the aging of the population, and adopt new technologies. These challenges and the transformation of the Medicaid program increase the importance of federal oversight and we stand ready to assist Congress in carrying out this oversight.

---

[19]See, for example, GAO, *Medicaid: Prototype Formula Would Provide Automatic, Targeted Assistance to States during Economic Downturns*, GAO-12-38 (Washington, D.C.: Nov. 10, 2011); and *Medicaid: Improving Responsiveness of Federal Assistance to States during Economic Downturns*, GAO-11-395 (Washington, D.C.: March 31, 2011).

[20]See GAO-12-38.

[21]See GAO, *Medicaid: Alternative Measures Could Be Used to Allocate Funding More Equitably*, GAO-13-434 (Washington, D.C.: May 10, 2013).

Chairman Pitts, Ranking Member Green, and Members of the
Subcommittee, this concludes our prepared statement. We would be
pleased to respond to any questions that you might have at this time.

GAO Contacts and Staff Acknowledgments	If you or your staff have any questions about this testimony, please contact Katherine M. Iritani at (202) 512-7114 or iritanik@gao.gov or Carolyn L. Yocom at (202) 512-7114 or yocomc@gao.gov. Contact points for our Offices of Congressional Relations and Public Affairs may be found on the last page of this statement. Individuals making key contributions to this testimony include Robert Copeland, Assistant Director; Kristen Joan Anderson; Robin Burke; Drew Long; Jasleen Modi; and Jessica Morris.

Appendix I: Matters for Congressional Consideration and Selected Medicaid-Related Recommendations, as of June 2015

The following table lists prior Medicaid-related matters for congressional consideration GAO has suggested.

Table 1: Matters for Congressional Consideration

GAO Report	Matters for Congressional Consideration
Medicaid: More Transparency of and Accountability for Supplemental Payments Are Needed. GAO-13-48, November 26, 2012	Congress should consider requiring the Centers for Medicare & Medicaid Services (CMS) to 1. improve state reporting of non-disproportionate share hospital (DSH) supplemental payments, including requiring annual reporting of payments made to individual facilities and other information that the agency determines is necessary to oversee non-DSH supplemental payments; 2. clarify permissible methods for calculating non-DSH supplemental payments; and 3. require states to submit an annual independent certified audit verifying state compliance with permissible methods for calculating non-DSH supplemental payments.
Medicaid: Prototype Formula Would Provide Automatic, Targeted Assistance to States during Economic Downturns. GAO-12-38, November 10, 2011	Congress could consider enacting a Federal Medical Assistance Percentage (FMAP) formula that is targeted for variable state Medicaid needs and provides automatic, timely, and temporary increased FMAP assistance in response to national economic downturns.
Medicaid Demonstration Waivers: Recent HHS Approvals Continue to Raise Cost and Oversight Concerns. GAO-08-87, January 31, 2008	Congress may wish to consider requiring increased attention to fiscal responsibility in the approval of Section 1115 Medicaid demonstrations by requiring the Department of Health and Human Services (HHS) to improve the demonstration review process through steps such as clarifying criteria for reviewing and approving states' proposed spending limits; better ensuring that valid methods are used to demonstrate budget neutrality; and documenting and making public material explaining the basis for any approvals.

Source: GAO. | GAO-15-746T

The following table lists selected Medicaid-related recommendations GAO has made to the Department of Health and Human Services that the agency has either not taken or has not completed steps to implement the recommendation.

Table 2: Selected Medicaid-Related Recommendations, as of June 2015

GAO Report	Recommendation
Medicaid: Additional Actions Needed to Help Improve Provider and Beneficiary Fraud Controls. GAO-15-313, May 14, 2015	The Centers for Medicare & Medicaid Services (CMS) should 1. issue guidance to states to better identify beneficiaries who are deceased; and 2. provide guidance to states on the availability of automated information through Medicare's enrollment database—the Provider Enrollment, Chain, and Ownership System (PECOS)—and full access to all pertinent PECOS information, such as ownership information, to help screen Medicaid providers more efficiently and effectively.
Medicaid Demonstrations: Approval Criteria and Documentation Need to Show How Spending Furthers Medicaid Objectives. GAO-15-239, April 13, 2015	The Department of Health and Human Services (HHS) should 1. issue criteria for assessing whether section 1115 expenditure authorities are likely to promote Medicaid objectives; 2. ensure the application of these criteria is documented in all HHS's approvals of section 1115 demonstrations, including those approving new or extending or modifying existing expenditure authorities, to inform internal and external stakeholders—including states, the public, and Congress—of the basis for the agency's determinations that approved expenditure authorities are likely to promote Medicaid objectives; 3. take steps to ensure that Medicaid demonstration approval documentation consistently provides assurances—such as through claiming protocols or the application template—that states will avoid duplicative spending by offsetting as appropriate all other federal revenues received when claiming federal Medicaid matching funds.
Medicaid: CMS Oversight of Provider Payments Is Hampered by Limited Data and Unclear Policy. GAO-15-322, April 10, 2015	CMS should 1. take steps to ensure that states report accurate provider specific payment data that include accurate unique national provider identifiers; 2. develop a policy establishing criteria for when such payments at the provider level are economical and efficient; and 3. once criteria are developed, develop a process for identifying and reviewing payments to individual providers in order to determine whether they are economical and efficient.
Medicaid Information Technology: CMS Supports Use of Program Integrity Systems but Should Require States to Determine Effectiveness. GAO-15-207, January 30, 2015	HHS should direct CMS to require states to measure quantifiable benefits, such as cost reductions or avoidance, achieved as a result of operating information systems to help prevent and detect improper payments.
Medicaid: Additional Federal Action Needed to Further Improper Third-Party Liability Efforts. GAO-15-208, January 28, 2015	HHS should direct CMS to 1. routinely monitor and share across all states information regarding key third-party liability efforts and challenges; and 2. provide guidance to states on their oversight of third-party liability efforts conducted by Medicaid managed care plans.

43

GAO Report	Recommendation
Medicaid Financing: States' Increased Reliance on Funds from Health Care Providers and Local Governments Warrants Improved CMS Data Collection. GAO-14-627, July 29, 2014	CMS should develop a data collection strategy that ensures that states report accurate and complete data on all sources of funds used to finance the nonfederal share of Medicaid payments.
Medicaid Program Integrity: Increased Oversight Needed to Ensure Integrity of Growing Managed Care Expenditures. GAO-14-341, May 19, 2014	CMS should 1. hold states accountable for Medicaid managed care program integrity by requiring states to conduct audits of payments to and by managed care organizations; and 2. update CMS's Medicaid managed care guidance on program integrity practices and effective handling of managed care organization recoveries.
Medicaid Demonstration Waivers: Approval Process Raises Cost Concerns and Lacks Transparency. GAO-13-384, June 25, 2013	HHS should update the agency's written budget neutrality policy to reflect actual criteria and processes used to develop and approve demonstration spending limits, and ensure the policy is readily available to state Medicaid directors and others.
Medicaid and CHIP: Reports for Monitoring Children's Health Care Services Need Improvement. GAO-11-293R, April 5, 2011	CMS should work with states to identify additional improvements that could be made to the CMS 416 annual reports, including options for reporting on the receipt of services separately for children in managed care and fee-for-service delivery models, while minimizing reporting burden, and for capturing information on the CMS 416 relating to children's receipt of treatment services for which they are referred.

Source: GAO. | GAO-15-748T

Related GAO Products

The following are selected GAO products pertinent to the key issues discussed in this statement. Other products may be found at GAO's website at www.gao.gov.

Access to Care

Children's Health Insurance: Information on Coverage of Services, Costs to Consumers, and Access to Care in CHIP and Other Sources of Insurance. GAO-14-40. Washington, D.C.: November 21, 2013.

Children's Mental Health: Concerns Remain about Appropriate Services for Children in Medicaid and Foster Care. GAO-13-15. Washington, D.C.: December 10, 2012.

Medicaid: States Made Multiple Program Changes, and Beneficiaries Generally Reported Access Comparable to Private Insurance. GAO-13-55. Washington, D.C.: November 15, 2012.

Medicaid and CHIP: Most Physicians Serve Covered Children but Have Difficulty Referring Them for Specialty Care. GAO-11-624. Washington, D.C.: June 30, 2011.

Medicaid and CHIP: Reports for Monitoring Children's Health Care Services Need Improvement. GAO-11-293R. Washington, D.C.: April 5, 2011.

Oral Health: Efforts Under Way to Improve Children's Access to Dental Services, but Sustained Attention Needed to Address Ongoing Concerns. GAO-11-96. Washington, D.C.: November 30, 2010.

Medicaid: State and Federal Actions Have Been Taken to Improve Children's Access to Dental Services, but Gaps Remain. GAO-09-723. Washington, D.C.: September 30, 2009.

Transparency and Oversight

Medicaid Demonstrations: Approval Criteria and Documentation Need to Show How Spending Furthers Medicaid Objectives. GAO-15-239. Washington, D.C.: April 13, 2015.

Medicaid: CMS Oversight of Provider Payments Is Hampered by Limited Data and Unclear Policy. GAO-15-322. Washington, D.C.: April 10, 2015.

Medicaid Financing: Questionnaire Data on States' Methods for Financing Medicaid Payments from 2008 through 2012. GAO-15-227SP. Washington, D.C.: March 13, 2015, an e-supplement to GAO-14-627.

Medicaid Demonstrations: HHS's Approval Process for Arkansas's Medicaid Expansion Waiver Raises Cost Concerns. GAO-14-689R. Washington, D.C.: August 8, 2014.

Medicaid Financing: States' Increased Reliance on Funds from Health Care Providers and Local Governments Warrants Improved CMS Data Collection. GAO-14-627. Washington, D.C.: July 29, 2014.

Medicaid Demonstration Waivers: Approval Process Raises Cost Concerns and Lacks Transparency. GAO-13-384. Washington, D.C.: June 25, 2013.

Medicaid: More Transparency of and Accountability for Supplemental Payments Are Needed. GAO-13-48. Washington, D.C.: November 26, 2012.

Medicaid: CMS Needs More Information on the Billions of Dollars Spent on Supplemental Payments. GAO-08-614. Washington, D.C.: May 30, 2008.

Medicaid Demonstration Waivers: Recent HHS Approvals Continue to Raise Cost and Oversight Concerns. GAO-08-87. Washington, D.C.: January 31, 2008.

Medicaid Financing: Federal Oversight Initiative Is Consistent with Medicaid Payment Principles but Needs Greater Transparency. GAO-07-214. Washington, D.C.: March 30, 2007.

Program Integrity

Medicaid: Additional Actions Needed to Help Improve Provider and Beneficiary Fraud Controls. GAO-15-313. Washington, D.C.: May 14, 2015.

Medicaid Information Technology: CMS Supports Use of Program Integrity Systems but Should Require States to Determine Effectiveness. GAO-15-207. Washington, D.C.: January 30, 2015.

Medicaid: Additional Federal Action Needed to Further Improve Third-Party Liability Efforts. GAO-15-208. Washington, D.C.: January 28, 2015.

46

|---|---|
Related GAO Products

Medicaid Program Integrity: Increased Oversight Needed to Ensure Integrity of Growing Managed Care Expenditures. GAO-14-341. Washington, D.C.: May 19, 2014.

Fraud Detection Systems: Centers for Medicare and Medicaid Services Needs to Ensure More Widespread Use. GAO-11-475. Washington, D.C.: June 30, 2011.

Federal Financing

Medicaid: Alternative Measures Could Be Used to Allocate Funding More Equitably. GAO-13-434. Washington, D.C.: May 10, 2013.

Medicaid: Prototype Formula Would Provide Automatic, Targeted Assistance to States during Economic Downturns. GAO-12-38. Washington, D.C.: November 10, 2011.

Medicaid: Improving Responsiveness of Federal Assistance to States during Economic Downturns. GAO-11-395. Washington, D.C.: March 31, 2011.

Other GAO Products

High-Risk Series: An Update. GAO-15-290. Washington, D.C.: February 11, 2015.

47

This is a work of the U.S. government and is not subject to copyright protection in the United States. The published product may be reproduced and distributed in its entirety without further permission from GAO. However, because this work may contain copyrighted images or other material, permission from the copyright holder may be necessary if you wish to reproduce this material separately.

GAO's Mission	The Government Accountability Office, the audit, evaluation, and investigative arm of Congress, exists to support Congress in meeting its constitutional responsibilities and to help improve the performance and accountability of the federal government for the American people. GAO examines the use of public funds; evaluates federal programs and policies; and provides analyses, recommendations, and other assistance to help Congress make informed oversight, policy, and funding decisions. GAO's commitment to good government is reflected in its core values of accountability, integrity, and reliability.
Obtaining Copies of GAO Reports and Testimony	The fastest and easiest way to obtain copies of GAO documents at no cost is through GAO's website (http://www.gao.gov). Each weekday afternoon, GAO posts on its website newly released reports, testimony, and correspondence. To have GAO e-mail you a list of newly posted products, go to http://www.gao.gov and select "E-mail Updates."
Order by Phone	The price of each GAO publication reflects GAO's actual cost of production and distribution and depends on the number of pages in the publication and whether the publication is printed in color or black and white. Pricing and ordering information is posted on GAO's website, http://www.gao.gov/ordering.htm. Place orders by calling (202) 512-6000, toll free (866) 801-7077, or TDD (202) 512-2537. Orders may be paid for using American Express, Discover Card, MasterCard, Visa, check, or money order. Call for additional information.
Connect with GAO	Connect with GAO on Facebook, Flickr, Twitter, and YouTube. Subscribe to our RSS Feeds or E-mail Updates. Listen to our Podcasts and read The Watchblog. Visit GAO on the web at www.gao.gov.
To Report Fraud, Waste, and Abuse in Federal Programs	Contact: Website: http://www.gao.gov/fraudnet/fraudnet.htm E-mail: fraudnet@gao.gov Automated answering system: (800) 424-5454 or (202) 512-7470
Congressional Relations	Katherine Siggerud, Managing Director, siggerudk@gao.gov, (202) 512-4400, U.S. Government Accountability Office, 441 G Street NW, Room 7125, Washington, DC 20548
Public Affairs	Chuck Young, Managing Director, youngc1@gao.gov, (202) 512-4800 U.S. Government Accountability Office, 441 G Street NW, Room 7149 Washington, DC 20548

Please Print on Recycled Paper.

49

Mr. PITTS. The Chair thanks the gentlelady. And, again, as noted, Ms. Yocom's accompanied by Ms. Iritani, who testified before us a couple of weeks ago. She is back to help answer questions for GAO.

The Chair now recognizes Dr. Schwartz, 5 minutes for an opening statement.

STATEMENT OF ANNE L. SCHWARTZ

Dr. SCHWARTZ. Good morning, Chairman Pitts, Ranking Member Green, and members of the Subcommittee on Health. I am Anne Schwartz, Executive Director of MACPAC, the Medicaid and CHIP Payment and Access Commission. As you know, MACPAC is a Congressional advisory body charged with analyzing and reviewing Medicaid and CHIP policies, and making recommendations to Congress, the Secretary of HHS, and the States on issues affecting these programs. Its 17 members, led by Chair Diane Rowland and Vice Chair Marsha Gold, are appointed by GAO. The insights I will share this morning reflect the consensus views of the Commission itself, and we appreciate the opportunity to share MACPAC's views as this committee considers the future of Medicaid.

As others have already noted, Medicaid is a major and important part of the U.S. healthcare system, covering 72 million people, and almost half of the Nation's births. It pays for more than 60 percent of national spending on long-term services and supports to frail elders and other people with disabilities, and it accounts for more than a quarter of spending on treatment for mental health and substance use disorders. In total, it accounts for about 15 percent of national health expenditures, 8.6 percent of Federal outlays, and 15.1 percent of State spending.

While we often compare Medicaid's performance as a payer with other sources of coverage, it is important to recognize Medicaid's unique roles. In addition to providing health insurance to individuals who otherwise might not have access to coverage, it is also a major source of revenue for safety net providers serving both Medicaid beneficiaries and the uninsured. It covers enabling services, such as nonemergency transportation and translation services, which help beneficiaries access needed health services, and it wraps around other sources of coverage, including both employer sponsored insurance and Medicare, in its role for 10.7 million dually eligible beneficiaries.

Since the early 1990s the Medicaid program has changed in significant ways. During this time period the country weathered two economic recessions, and States responded to budgetary pressures by undertaking modernization efforts and cost containment strategies. As a result, as has been noted, managed care has now become the dominant delivery system, with more than half of all beneficiaries enrolled in comprehensive risk-based managed care arrangements, and another 20 percent receiving benefits through a more limited managed care arrangement.

The Olmstead Decision, requiring that people with disabilities be served in the least restrictive environment, resulted in a major shift in the provision of long-term services and supports from nursing facilities to home and community-based settings. Congressional action in the 1990s brought in children's coverage through Medicaid and CHIP, and encouraged States to reach out to people who are eligible, but not enrolled in coverage. And, of course, more recently the Affordable Care Act created new dynamics not just by allowing States to expand coverage to certain nondisabled adults, but also by providing new options to States for the delivery of home and community-based services, and by changing eligibility processes to allow for one-stop shopping for individuals seeking healthcare coverage.

The 20 years ahead are likely to be similarly dynamic as States experiment with different approaches to delivery system reform and payment, and seek to provide care more efficiently and effectively to high cost, high need individuals. Pressure on Federal and State budgets create challenges to ensuring the sustainability of the program, as well as to ensuring that beneficiaries have access to high value services that promote their health and their ability to function in their communities.

MACPAC's analytic agenda for the year ahead reflects several of these challenges. We will extend the work published in our recent June report on Medicaid's role for people with behavioral health disorders, focusing on how to improve delivery of care. We will continue to focus on understanding the impact of value-based purchasing initiatives, and the extent to which these bend the cost curve and improve health.

In the area of access, we will be determining how to effectively measure access and looking closely at the extent to which different groups of Medicaid beneficiaries are at risk of access barriers, and the extent to which such barriers can be addressed through Medicaid policy. Our analyses on the impact of the ACA will include, at the request of Congress, a study to model the impact of DSH payment cuts, and we will also consider how different approaches to Medicaid expansion affect expenditures and use of services. At the request of members of this committee and others in Congress, we will analyze spending trends and evaluate policy options to restructure the program's financing, and we will be moving ahead to the next chapter of our work on children's coverage, looking ahead before CHIP funding expires in fiscal year 2017.

Finally, we will continue to highlight the importance of having timely and complete data for both policy analysis and program accountability. MACPAC has also expressed concerns about administrative capacity constraints that affect the ability of both Federal and State administrators to meet program requirements, provide oversight, and promote value to beneficiaries, and to the taxpayer.

Again, thank you for this opportunity to share the Commission's work with the subcommittee, and I am happy to answer any questions.

[The prepared statement of Ms. Schwartz follows:]

MACPAC

Advising Congress on
Medicaid and CHIP Policy

Statement of
Anne L. Schwartz, Ph.D., Executive Director

Medicaid and CHIP
Payment and Access Commission

Before the
Subcommittee on Health
House Committee on Energy and Commerce

July 8, 2015

Medicaid and CHIP Payment
and Access Commission

1800 M Street NW
Suite 650 South
Washington, DC 20036

www.macpac.gov
202-350-2000
202-273-2452

52

Summary

Medicaid is a major part of the U.S. health care system, covering 72 million people, almost half of the nation's births, and paying for more than 60 percent of long-term services and supports (LTSS), and more than a quarter of treatment for mental health and substance use disorders. It accounts for about 15 percent of national health spending, 8.6 percent of federal outlays, and 15.1 percent of state spending.

While we often compare Medicaid's performance with other sources of coverage, it is important to recognize its unique roles. It provides health insurance to individuals who otherwise may not have access to coverage and is a major source of revenue for safety net providers serving both Medicaid beneficiaries and the uninsured. It covers LTSS and enabling services which help beneficiaries access needed health services, and wraps around other sources of coverage, including employer-sponsored insurance and Medicare.

Since the early 1990s, the Medicaid program has changed in significant ways. During this time period, the country weathered two economic recessions. States responded by undertaking modernization efforts and cost containment strategies. Managed care is now the dominant delivery system with about half of all beneficiaries enrolled in comprehensive risk-based plans. The Olmstead decision requiring that persons with disabilities be served in the least restrictive environment resulted in a major shift in the provision of LTSS from nursing facilities to home and community-based settings. Congressional action in the 1990s broadened children's coverage through Medicaid and the State Children's Health Insurance Program (CHIP), and encouraged states to reach out to people eligible but not enrolled in coverage. More recently, the Patient Protection and Affordable Care Act (ACA, P.L. 111-148, as amended) created new dynamics, allowing states to expand coverage to certain non-disabled adults, as well as providing new delivery system options to states and allowing for one-stop shopping for individuals seeking health care coverage.

The 20 years ahead are likely to be similarly dynamic as states experiment with new approaches to delivery system design and provider payment, and seek to provide care more effectively and efficiently for high-cost, high-need individuals, such as those with behavioral health conditions and beneficiaries who are dually eligible for Medicare and Medicaid. Pressure on federal and state budgets create challenges to ensuring both the sustainability of the program and that beneficiaries have access to high-value services that promote their health and ability to function in their communities.

MACPAC's analytic agenda for the year ahead reflects these challenges. We will extend our work on Medicaid's role for people with behavioral health disorders, focusing on how to improve the delivery of care. We will continue to focus on understanding the impact of value-based purchasing initiatives and the extent to which these bend the cost curve and improve health. In the area of access, we will examine how to effectively measure access, the extent to which different groups of beneficiaries are at risk of access barriers, and the extent to which such barriers can be addressed through Medicaid policy. Our analyses on the impact of the ACA will, as required by Congress, model the impact of disproportionate share hospital payment reductions. At the request of members of this committee and others in Congress, we will analyze and evaluate various policy options to restructure the program's financing. We will move to the next chapter in our work on children's coverage, looking ahead to recommend policies to assure adequate and affordable coverage for low- and moderate income children before CHIP funding expires in FY 2017. Finally we will continue to highlight the importance of having appropriate data for both policy analysis and program accountability. MACPAC has also commented on administrative capacity constraints that affect the ability of federal and state administrators to meet program requirements, provide oversight, promote value, and integrate Medicaid and CHIP into broader delivery system and financing reforms.

● ● ✹

Medicaid and CHIP Payment
and Access Commission
www.macpac.gov

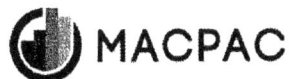 MACPAC

Statement of Anne L. Schwartz, Ph.D., Executive Director
Medicaid and CHIP Payment and Access Commission

Good morning Chairman Pitts, Ranking Member Green, and Members of the Subcommittee on Health. I am Anne Schwartz, executive director of MACPAC, the Medicaid and CHIP Payment and Access Commission.

As you know, MACPAC is a congressional advisory body charged with analyzing and reviewing Medicaid and State Children's Health Insurance Program (CHIP) policies and making recommendations to Congress, the Secretary of the U.S. Department of Health and Human Services, and the states on issues affecting these programs. Its 17 members, led by Chair Diane Rowland and Vice Chair Marsha Gold, are appointed by the U.S. Government Accountability Office. The insights and expertise I will share this morning reflect the consensus views of the Commission itself. We appreciate the opportunity to share MACPAC's recommendations and work as this committee considers the future of Medicaid.

Medicaid is a major and important part of the U.S. health care system, covering 72 million people in fiscal year (FY) 2013, more than 20 percent of the U.S. population. The program covers almost half of the nation's births, pays for more than 60 percent of national spending on long-term services and supports (LTSS) to frail elders and other people with disabilities, and accounts for more than a quarter of national spending on treatment for mental health and substance use disorders. In total, it accounts for about 15 percent of national health expenditures, 8.6 percent of federal outlays, and 15.1 percent of spending from state-funded budgets, including state general funds, bonds, and other state funds (which for Medicaid includes provider taxes and local funds that flow through the

Medicaid and CHIP Payment
and Access Commission

1800 M Street NW
Suite 650 South
Washington, DC 20036

www.macpac.gov
202-350-2000 ☎
202-273-2452 📠

54

state budget). It should be noted that while Medicaid has grown as a share of the federal budget, increasing from 1.4 percent of federal outlays in FY 1970 to 8.6 percent in FY 2014, annual growth in Medicaid spending per enrollee has been lower or comparable to Medicare and private insurance since the early 1990s.

While we often compare Medicaid's performance as a payer with other sources of coverage, such as Medicare and employer-sponsored insurance, it is important to recognize Medicaid's unique roles. In addition to providing health insurance to individuals who otherwise may not have access to coverage, it is also a major source of revenue for safety net providers serving both Medicaid beneficiaries and those without insurance. It covers enabling services such as non-emergency transportation and translation services that help beneficiaries access needed health services. Moreover, it wraps around other sources of coverage, including both employer-sponsored insurance and Medicare in its role for 10.7 million dually eligible beneficiaries. Notably, despite the fact that Medicare is the major source of medical coverage for the nation's elderly, it does not cover LTSS. For those in need of long-term care, Medicaid coverage for ongoing nursing facility or other institutional arrangements, home health, personal care, and other home and community-based services (HCBS) is vital to their daily lives.

Looking Back

Since the early 1990s, the Medicaid program has changed in significant ways. During this time period, the country weathered two economic recessions. States responded to budgetary pressures by undertaking modernization efforts and cost containment strategies. As a result, the program has moved from a traditional fee-for-service model to one in which managed care has become the dominant delivery system. More than half of all beneficiaries are now enrolled in comprehensive risk-based plans, and another 20 percent receive some of their benefits through a non-comprehensive managed care arrangement, including primary care case management and limited benefit plans. While initially managed care covered primarily children and their mothers, increasingly managed care is being extended to populations with more complex health needs. Managed care is also transforming the delivery of long-term services and supports. In 2004, just eight states had managed LTSS programs. By the end of this year, more than half of the states are expected to be using managed care models for such services.

The Supreme Court's 1999 decision in *Olmstead v. L.C.* requiring that persons with disabilities be served in the least restrictive environment resulted in a major shift in the provision of long-term services and supports from nursing facilities to home and community-based settings. In FY 1995, 18 percent of Medicaid LTSS spending occurred in a non-institutional setting; by FY 2012, the figure had risen to nearly half.

In the 1990s, congressional action broadened children's coverage through Medicaid and CHIP, and encouraged states to reach out to people eligible but not enrolled in coverage. These actions substantially reduced the share of children without health insurance. In 1997, 22.4 percent of children below the federal poverty level and 22.8 percent of those with family incomes between 100 and 200 percent FPL were uninsured. By 2014, these percentages had dropped to 6.9 percent and 8.9 percent respectively.

More recently, the Patient Protection and Affordable Care Act (ACA, P.L. 111-148, as amended) created new dynamics, allowing states to expand coverage to previously ineligible childless adults and parents. Twenty nine states and the District of Columbia have now expanded their programs, and other states are examining their options. Streamlined eligibility and enrollment processes, including the adoption of modified adjusted gross income (MAGI) as the standard for income determinations, now allow for one-stop shopping for individuals seeking health care coverage. The law also created new options for states for delivery of HCBS, including the Community First Choice program for individuals who are eligible for Medicaid and have incomes below 150 percent FPL but who may not meet institutional level-of-care criteria, or those with such needs whose incomes exceed 150 percent FPL, the Health Homes option, extension and modification of the Money Follows the Person demonstration, and establishment of the state Balancing Incentive Payments program.

Looking Ahead

The 20 years ahead are likely to be similarly dynamic as states experiment with different approaches to delivery system design and payment, including the delivery system reform incentive payment (DSRIP) programs described in MACPAC's June 2015 report to Congress. States are also seeking to provide care more effectively and efficiently for high-cost, high-need individuals such as those with behavioral health conditions and beneficiaries dually eligible for Medicare and Medicaid, also the subject of analysis in our 2015 reports.

Pressure on federal and state budgets creates challenges to ensuring the sustainability of the program and making certain that beneficiaries have access to high-value services that promote their health and ability to function in their communities. These challenges are not unique to Medicaid. Between FY 2014 and FY 2022, annual growth in Medicaid spending per enrollee is projected to average about 4 percent, similar to the rate for Medicare and lower than the rate for private insurance.

MACPAC's Agenda

●●●
Medicaid and CHIP Payment
and Access Commission
www.macpac.gov

MACPAC's analytic agenda for the year ahead reflects several of these challenges. We will extend the work published in our June report on Medicaid's role for people with behavioral health disorders, focusing on how to improve the delivery of care and better understand models of integration for various subpopulations such as those with serious mental illness. We will also continue to focus on the impact of value-based purchasing initiatives including accountable care organizations, bundled payments, and patient-centered medical homes, and the extent to which these bend the cost curve and improve health.

In the area of access, we will be strengthening and extending our longstanding efforts to measure access to care, an issue now more salient than ever given the Supreme Court's decision in *Armstrong v. Exceptional Child Center* which will put new pressures on the federal government to ensure that Medicaid payment rates are sufficient to ensure access comparable to that of the general population. In addition, we will be examining more closely the extent to which different groups of Medicaid beneficiaries are at risk of access barriers and for which services (for example, specialty care) and the extent to which such barriers can be effectively addressed through Medicaid policy.

Our analyses on the impact of the ACA will include a major effort, as required by Congress, to model the impact of disproportionate share hospital (DSH) payment reductions. Our first report examining the impact that such changes will have on hospitals is due February 1st of next year. In addition, building on our March 2015 report chapter examining premium assistance models in Arkansas and Iowa, we will be also be considering how different approaches to Medicaid expansion affect expenditures and use of services.

●●○
Medicaid and CHIP Payment
and Access Commission
www.macpac.gov

At the request of members of this committee and others in Congress, we will analyze and evaluate various policy options to restructure the program's financing. We will be moving to the next chapter in our work on children's coverage, looking ahead to recommend what policies should be in place to assure adequate and affordable coverage for low- and moderate-income children before CHIP funding expires in FY 2017.

Finally we will continue to highlight the importance of having appropriate data available for both policy analysis and program accountability. Since its inaugural report to Congress in March 2011, the Commission has continually called for improvements in the timeliness, quality, and availability of administrative data on Medicaid and CHIP, noting the importance of these data in answering key policy and operational questions that affect beneficiaries, providers, states, and the federal government. As noted in our June 2013 report, given that plans to modernize federal data systems currently rely on a patchwork of program integrity, quality measurement, health information technology, and CHIP reauthorization funds, the Commission is concerned whether available resources are sufficient for this purpose.

MACPAC has also commented on administrative capacity constraints at the federal and state levels that affect the ability to meet program requirements, provide oversight, and take on broader delivery system reforms that promote value and contain costs. As noted in the Commission's June 2014 report, there are few clear performance standards or metrics to assess state capacity, identify gaps in performance, prioritize investments, and identify appropriate responses. This is an area where we plan to work with state officials and experts in performance management to shed light on promising approaches.

● ● ⬤

Medicaid and CHIP Payment
and Access Commission
www.macpac.gov

Again, thank you for this opportunity to share the Commission's work with this subcommittee and I am happy to

answer any questions.

● ● ◇
Medicaid and CHIP Payment
and Access Commission
www.macpac.gov

Mr. PITTS. The Chair thanks the gentlelady. That concludes the opening statements. We will begin questioning, and I will recognize myself for 5 minutes for that purpose.

Ms. Wachino, the part of the Federal statute on the 1115 waivers is very short, just four pages. So the Secretary of HHS has tremendous latitude under the law to fund some demonstration projects, while denying others. It is well known that some States get CMS approval for a specific proposal, while CMS will deny another State for a very similar proposal. My first question is, Are there any statutory criteria requiring consistency related to the Secretary's review and approval of demonstration projects?

Ms. WACHINO. Chairman, thank you for the question. CMS works with all States in the 1115 process, and outside of it, to develop approaches that meet the objectives of the Medicaid program, and take into account State-specific needs in surveying and meeting the needs of their low-income population. We approach that process consistently across States, and we work with each State to identify the extent to which their proposal meets the objectives of the program, and improves the health of lower/low-income residents.

We have been very transparent in our decision-making on 1115s. We issued transparency regulations implementing provisions to the Affordable Care Act several years ago, and have been posting all of our approval documents on medicaid.gov for States to see, and we welcome proposals from additional States, and will consider them on their merits.

Mr. PITTS. The question was, are there any statutory criteria requiring consistency?

Ms. WACHINO. The statutory criterion is that a proposal meet the objectives of the Medicaid program.

Mr. PITTS. Does CMS have regulations or guidance to ensure that it is being consistent and equitable?

Ms. WACHINO. We have guidance implementing our transparency requirements. Those were regulations that were implemented in 2012. We identified, subsequent to the GAO report, broad criteria that we used in considering every State's waiver to determine whether it meets the objectives of the Medicaid program, and those were criteria like expanding access to coverage, strengthening delivery systems. So, yes, we have developed a set of principles by which we review 1115 demonstrations.

It is also important to us, though, to be able to take into account State-specific circumstances. States come to us with a wide array of proposals, and if you look across waivers you will see that they serve purposes as diverse as expanding eligibility to new populations, to providing limited benefits, like prescription drugs, to reforming State delivery systems.

Mr. PITTS. Dr. Schwartz, in April several chairmen of the committees of jurisdiction sent you a letter requesting that MACPAC undertake serious and sustained analytical work to advise Congress about potential policies and needed financing reforms and incentives to ensure the sustainability of Medicaid. Can you please explain to the committee, in specific detail, how you are responding to that request, and when you—we can expect to start seeing the results of your work?

Dr. SCHWARTZ. Yes. Since the Commission received the letter in April, we have had one public meeting in May. At that May meeting we presented analyses that were already underway on Federal and State spending trends that we are currently turning into a publication that should be out later this summer.

We are now currently determining our next agenda for the next report cycle, bringing to fruition work on understanding innovative approaches that States are taking to build more sustainable programs. For example, the use of accountable care organization, bundled payments, patient-centered medical homes, managed long-term services and supports, and trying to look at these designs and see what the potential is for savings in both the short and the long term.

Specifically to the items mentioned in your letter, we do have analyses underway to review the past work of blue ribbon commissions and think tanks so as not to reinvent the wheel, and we will use those to inform our analyses of technical and design issues associated with some of those proposals, as well as more recent approaches that have been put forward by members of this committee and others.

So the letter speaks to a sustained work plan, and you can expect to see some of this work coming together over the course of the fall to inform our March and June reports, and follow-ons after that. Mr. PITTS. Thank you. Ms. Wachino, has CMS determined an eligibility error rate for the Obamacare expansion population, and how does the error rate vary for those determined Medicaid eligible through the Federally facilitated marketplace versus those whom States determine eligibility?

Ms. WACHINO. Mr. Chairman, within CMS there are other parts of the organization that have responsibility for the error rate measurement. I can say that I know that we have piloted approaches to measuring eligibility errors with States in order to ensure that we are measuring eligibility effectively as we move to the new rules under the ACA, and we would be happy to get back to you with a report out for the record on what we know from those pilots so far.

Mr. PITTS. Thank you. My time is expired. The Chair recognizes the ranking member, Mr. Green, 5 minutes for questions.

Mr. GREEN. Thank you, Mr. Chairman. This year marks the 50th anniversary of Medicaid. It is a vital program that is served as a lifeline for millions of Americans that—when they need it the most. It is important to recognize the successes that it made, innovations that are working well, and improvements that could be implemented. We have seen some outstanding success ensuring the overwhelming majority of Medicaid beneficiaries have access to primary care. More than 95 percent of the Medicaid beneficiaries not only have access to primary care, but are satisfied with that care.

The committee has made substantial investments in the Community Health Center Program, particularly when it comes to grant funding intended to cover the uninsured. One aspect that is not talked about as frequently is that of the unique role and intertwined nature of community health centers and Medicaid.

Ms. Wachino, could CMS comment on the role that community health centers, and—a crucial source of primary care have played to bring along—about the level of success of Medicaid beneficiaries?

Ms. WACHINO. Thank you for the question. Community centers play a really vital role in serving our populations and meeting the needs of a diverse range of Americans, particularly focused on pri- mary care. Community health centers are playing a growing role in meeting low-income Americans' oral healthcare needs, which are important to us, and we continue to work with them to make their payment systems as strong as possible.

Mr. GREEN. OK. Thank you. And I know we still have work to do on—to ensure equal access to dental and specialty care. In par- ticular, access to behavioral health providers is an issue this com- mittee has considered, and all three of our witnesses know well.

Ms. Wachino, CMS is working hard with States to promote inno- vative care delivery, integrating physical and mental health, or promoting oral health, as part of the comprehensive primary care. Can you provide the committee with a few examples of how CMS work on Medicaid delivery system reform is helping to promote ac- cess to these specialty providers?

Ms. WACHINO. Sure, I would be happy to, thank you. Through our Innovation Accelerator Program, which, as I mentioned earlier, is our new delivery system reform initiative aimed at providing program support to States that would like to improve their pay- ment and delivery system, we identified four areas that were estab- lished with the input of States and stakeholders that were prior- ities of our program, substance use disorder, physical and behav- ioral health integration, community integration, moving away from institutional care to community care, and meeting the needs of complex, high cost beneficiaries.

The first two I think, Ranking Member Green, are responsive to your question. And the area in which we have done the most work so far in this new program is substance use disorder, and we are working actively right now with seven States to help expand the range of providers who can provide substance use disorder sup- ports, and we expect to bring a similar approach to physical and behavioral health to really help ensure that there is access to com- munity-based mental health services for the people who need it.

Mr. GREEN. OK. I was impressed to see provisions on adequate— or quality and actuarial soundness and network adequacy in the new Medicaid managed care regulation. Can you describe how, if CMS' proposed managed care regulation would be implemented, ac- cess to quality care would improve beneficiaries in the managed care?

Ms. WACHINO. Sure. I will highlight a couple of examples of how our new proposed rule could improve quality and actuarial sound- ness and access for our populations. With regard to quality, there are a number of provisions. I think one of the most significant is giving Medicaid beneficiaries the ability to understand how quality compares across plans through a new quality rating system, so that beneficiaries can shop, and they can form choices about their plan selections.

As you referred to, Ranking Member Green, we also substantially have improved our approach to ensuring that plan rates are actuarially sound. There is a body of work reviewing those rates that is going on now, even in advance of the regulation, to really make sure that we are paying the right amount to ensure adequate access to Medicaid beneficiaries, and ensuring appropriate steward-ship of funds.

And with respect particularly to access, the proposed rule estab-lishes for the first time—or proposes to establish that there will be State-developed network adequacy standards for many key services for the Medicaid population, which, given that, as recently as 3 years ago, nearly 60 percent of our beneficiaries were enrolled in managed care, I think is a really substantial advance in access for our program.

Mr. GREEN. OK. Mr. Chairman, I have one last question for Ms. Schwartz. Has MACPAC looked at how changes to streamline eligi-bility have improved the continuity of care?

Dr. SCHWARTZ. We have not specifically analyzed that issue. It is one we are very interested in, and the data are not yet available for us to do so. And as data become available, that is something that we will be keeping our eye on.

Mr. PITTS. The Chair thanks the gentleman. I recognize the chair emeritus of the full committee, Mr. Barton, 5 minutes for ques-tions.

Mr. BARTON. Thank you, Mr. Chairman, and thank you for the hearing. These microphones kind of have an echo to them. I will be as softly as I can.

Ms. Wachino, could you give us the status of the Texas request for re-approval of its 1115 waiver?

Ms. WACHINO. Yes, I can. The Texas waiver expires next year. I know that the State has been working on a request to extend that demonstration, which we approved in 2011, but they have not sent it to us yet. We have had some initial conversations with them, but are waiting for them to submit their full request, and look forward to working with them on it.

Mr. BARTON. So there have been some rumors that because Texas is such a red State that that application is going to be frowned upon. That is just rumors? There is no validity to that?

Ms. WACHINO. Congressman Barton, we work with all States through the waiver process to try to achieve the objectives of the Medicaid program and try to take into account State-specific needs, and we are looking forward to reviewing with the State of Texas how the initial demonstration went. There were some areas of their programs that were new to us when we initially approved it. We will want to review very closely with them how the different provi-sions of the waiver are working. And we are looking forward to that discussion.

Mr. BARTON. With Mr. Green here, my ally, make sure we are bipartisan, you will——

Mr. GREEN. Would you yield to me just for a minute?

Mr. BARTON. I will be happy to yield.

Mr. GREEN. Even though we are a red State, we sure have a lot of poor people, and Medicaid is for that, whether you are red or blue, or——

Mr. BARTON. That is true.

Mr. GREEN [continuing]. Whatever. Thank you, Joe, for your leadership on what we are trying to do.

Mr. BARTON. Of course, those of us that are red, in that sense, you know, if they would listen to us more, we would have less of those people. See, we would get them into where they didn't need to be a part of it, but that is a different discussion.

So we have your word that the Texas 1115 waiver application is going to be fairly reviewed?

Ms. WACHINO. Again, we work with all States, you know, and we apply the same process to all States. We look to review the extent to which a waiver achieves the objectives of the Medicaid program and how it is advancing the health of the low-income population in the State. And I——

Mr. BARTON. So that is a yes?

Ms. WACHINO. I know that the team in Texas is working hard, and we are looking forward to working with them.

Mr. BARTON. OK. I am going to take that as a yes. We are going to put it in the record as a yes, that it is going to be fairly reviewed.

Let us look at a program, Ms.—that Ms. Castor and I are very supportive of, the Ace Kids Act. It would allow States to set up programs across State lines for special needs children, create a medical home in these anchor children's hospitals, where a parent could bring a child, and if the child qualifies, they get the full range of services, whatever those services need to be. This is a bipartisan bill. We have got—I can't remember how many co-sponsors, but it is well over 100. Are you familiar with that bill?

Ms. WACHINO. Congressman Barton, I can't say that I have looked at the particulars of that bill, but clearly approaches that advance the quality of care and coordination of care for children particularly are of interest to us, so I am happy to take a look at it, and CMS stands ready to provide any technical assistance to you on it.

Mr. BARTON. Well, the advocates of it, and I am an advocate for it, believe that it would save money for Medicaid. You wouldn't have to have a parent try to create their own network, and in some States you don't even have the type of care that that child needs. So it has got a lot of support, and I would encourage you and your staff to take a look at it, and hopefully, at the appropriate time, be supportive of it. And with that, Mr. Chairman, I yield back.

Mr. PITTS. The Chair thanks the gentleman. I now recognize the gentlelady from California, Mrs. Capps, 5 minutes for questions.

Mrs. CAPPS. Thank you, Mr. Chairman, and I appreciate the presence of our witnesses today, and your testimony. It is very appropriate that we are here during this anniversary year to talk about the largest source of health coverage in our country, Medicaid, and the Children's Health Insurance Program, CHIP. These programs now provide health care—or opportunities for health for over 70 million Americans, and I am happy that our committee was able to ensure that CHIP is re-authorized for 2 more years, and I hope that we continue to actively support and ensure the continuation of something I have known, as a school nurse, as an incredibly successful program.

As a committee, we have a responsibility to make our best faith effort to build upon the success of these programs. First, it is important to recognize how far the Medicaid program has come in the last 50 years. It is remarkable. Perhaps most notably, in the past few years, the program has been very much strengthened through the provisions in the Affordable Care Act based on the needs of our communities.

Medicaid is a safety net, of course, for these people who are otherwise shut out of private insurance, either because it is unaffordable, or is unavailable to them. And thanks to Medicaid expansion in the States where they have access to it, the program could be there for any of us, including here, in this room, who fall down on our luck and needed support.

Most people in the coverage gap are working. They are working poor, employed either part time or full time, but still living below the property line. While the promise of coverage is there, unfortunately, nearly four million hard-working low-income Americans cannot receive the health coverage they need because they live in States that have chosen not to expand Medicaid, despite the economic benefits that are now demonstrated, well demonstrated, of doing so. However, for those who do have Medicaid coverage, there have been substantial changes to the delivery of Medicaid that aim to increase access, and also quality of care. I am particularly proud of all the progress in my home State of California made in the areas of patient-centered medical homes and care coordination.

This has been discussed by you already in a response to a question, but can you talk about, Ms. Wachino, some of the other new and innovative delivery system reforms that you have seen States starting to take up, and have been working with States to make sure it happens?

Ms. WACHINO. Sure, I am happy to, thank you. We have a variety of really promising work underway with States to strengthen their delivery systems. And, as I said briefly in my oral testimony, there are many different modalities.

Mrs. CAPPS. Um-hum.

Ms. WACHINO. Some States, you know, use existing State plan authority. States like Arkansas are taking up shared savings for their providers, building off of a Medicare model. Missouri is using our new health homes option, created under the Affordable Care Act, to really move forward with improvements for people with chronic diseases. And in Missouri we have seen reductions in the use of hospital care, and improvements in key measures, like measures of diabetes care, which are very, very promising.

There are other States who have taken even more far-reaching approaches. Oregon, under 1115 authority several years ago, launched coordinated care organizations, which were designed to be community rooted approaches to coordinating the entire spectrum of care for Medicaid beneficiaries and piloting new approaches, like using community health workers. Other States have created delivery system reform incentive payments to really propel movement forward on key payment goals. We approved New York last year for a new 1115 waiver, and New York is committed to very concrete and measurable objectives for increasing the number of their providers who are using value-based payments.

66

Mrs. CAPPS. Thank you.

Ms. WACHINO. So I think we are changing the landscape of Medicaid care delivery in a number of ways.

Mrs. CAPPS. I don't mean to cut you off, but I think you could go on and on, and maybe you would like——

Ms. WACHINO. I am afraid I can, so I thank you for the stop.

Mrs. CAPPS. You could submit any other examples you would like for the record, because, as we have discussed in this community 2 weeks ago, we have seen over 300 State flexibility waivers to create State solutions within the Medicaid framework. And that—this is an exciting time to see those come forward. There is substantial State flexibility. I think it is important to recognize this innovation and flexibility, what it looks like. Before considering any changes to our program, we must be mindful about what exactly—who will be impacted by the decisions that we might make, and if we are truly improving care, or just passing the buck to States.

So we want to be working with you—with the different States with respect to persons with disabilities, seniors, and struggling families. Right now we know that the Medicaid program works. Individuals with Medicaid are more likely to receive preventative health care, which is cost savings, and less likely to have medical debt than their underinsured counterparts.

Dr. Schwartz—I will have to save that question for another panel—another round. Thank you.

Mr. PITTS. Or you can submit it in writing. Thank you. The Chair thanks the gentlelady. I now recognize the vice chair of the subcommittee, Mr. Guthrie, 5 minutes for questions.

Mr. GUTHRIE. Hey, thank you. Thank you all for coming this morning. And, first, to either Ms. Yocom or Ms. Iritani, I hope I said that correctly, in your testimony you noted that CMS lacked complete and reliable data about the sources of funding States used to finance the non-Federal share of Medicaid, which can shift costs to the Federal Government. What information have you recommended that CMS collect, and how will having this information help CMS monitor the program to ensure the appropriate use of Federal funds?

Ms. IRITANI. Yes, we have made recommendations that CMS develop a data collection strategy regarding sources of funds that States use for financing the non-Federal share. We have recently surveyed States about how they are financing the non-Federal share, and identified that States are relying more heavily on providers, such as through provider taxes, and local governments, through intergovernmental transfers, for example.

Provider taxes, I think, doubled during the course of the 2008 to 2012 time period that we looked at, and these can shift costs to the Federal Government and to providers. We think it is important that CMS have data needed for oversight.

Mr. GUTHRIE. OK, thank you. And, Ms. Wachino, I have introduced a bill H.R. 1362, which would require States to report how they finance. I know you share that we need more transparency in the way States report how they finance Medicaid. And what actions has CMS taken in response to the GAO recommendations?

Ms. WACHINO. Mr. Guthrie, thank you for the question, and for your interest in transparency and accountability. I think GAO's work in this area has been very helpful, and we are making improvements, and continue to make more. We are looking much more closely at the sources, and reviewing more closely the sources of the non-Federal share. We are working on getting additional levels of data for a variety of different kinds of payments, and we are conducting more active oversight. We have also issued several forms of guidance to States, making sure that our rules are clear with respect to provider taxes and donations. So I think we are strong in this area, and continue to get stronger.

Mr. GUTHRIE. Yes, and I used to be in State Government, before I got here on the Budget Committee, in Kentucky, which has a substantial Medicaid population. Actually one out of four now are on Medicaid, and so I understand that States are being creative because of the budget pressures they are facing, so that is something we all need to work together to move forward.

And, Ms. Wachino, in your written statement you described numerous CMS initiatives aimed at innovation in achieving better health outcomes at a lower cost. And how is CMS assessing these— or evaluating these initiatives to determine if they are meeting goals?

Ms. WACHINO. A lot of these delivery system reforms are very important to us, and we want to know how they work for ourselves, as stewards of taxpayer dollars, and also to inform developments in other States. We are evaluating many of the delivery system reform improvements that we undertook with States through our 1115 waivers. Right now that is very important to us. MACPAC's also done some very helpful work in this area. And we also will be evaluating the effectiveness and results of the work we are doing through our Innovation Accelerator Program in areas like substance use disorder, promoting community integration, improving physical and behavioral health, and meeting the needs of complex, high cost populations. And, again, all of that is designed to help us, and to help States be smarter and better purchasers of care.

Mr. GUTHRIE. Well, good. Is there some timeframe when some of the original—or early evaluations will come forward?

Ms. WACHINO. You know, I can get back to you on that question for the record.

Mr. GUTHRIE. All right, thanks. And then one more. I understand that OIG has found significant and persistent compliance, payment, and fraud vulnerabilities related to the provision of personal care services in Medicaid, and—including payments for services not rendered. Has CMS taken action to address the OIG recommendations to improve integrity in personal care services?

Ms. WACHINO. Yes. Thank you for the question, and for the work that IG and GAO have done looking at our personal care services. We have taken steps to ensure the integrity of personal care services. We recently engaged a contractor to look at data and provider compliance——

Mr. GUTHRIE. Um-hum.

Ms. WACHINO [continuing]. In that area. We issued a quality informational bulletin with respect to personal care services in our 1915(c), which, apologies for the jargon, are home and community-based services waivers. And also, as I think staff of this committee knows, we have made a very substantial effort in data systems modernization. We call it our TMSIS System, and that is going to provide us a level of programmatic data that we are very eager for, and will help our program integrity, program management, ability to evaluate States in a number of areas, including for personal care services.

Mr. GUTHRIE. Thank you, my time has expired. I appreciate your answers. Appreciate your answers.

Mr. PITTS. The Chair thanks the gentleman. I now recognize the gentlelady from Florida, Ms. Castor, 5 minutes for questions.

Ms. CASTOR. Well, thank you, Mr. Chairman, and thank you to all of our witnesses for being here today to discuss Medicare on its 50th anniversary. You know, the passage of Medicare and Medicaid 50 years ago, through amendments to the Social Security Act, really are something to celebrate. They are landmark safety net laws in this country that really demonstrate our values. In Medicare, you work hard all of your life, and you retire, you are not going to fall into poverty because of a health condition. The same with Medicaid. Under Medicaid, we are not going to allow children across America, no matter what station they are born in in life, to suffer the consequences of a debilitating disability, or just being able to see a doctor.

So we have something to celebrate here. And then when you add on the impact of the Affordable Care Act, feels like we are kind of out of the woods, and now we can begin to work on bipartisan solutions to improve it together. I think the future is bright so—this is also an important time for Medicaid, because at this point in time we are dealing with Medicaid expansion and delivery system reform, and that will help improve the lives of so many of our neighbors all across the country. So I look forward to hearing your thoughts on these transformations.

I want to especially thank Ms. Wachino for her extensive work with the State of Florida over the past few months, few years. We had a very contentious legislative session, where we had Republican State Senators, and the business community, hospitals, clamoring for a coverage model in Medicaid expansion. We had a Governor who flip-flopped. He was for Medicaid expansion when he ran for re-election, then he changed after the election. He devised a budget with certain low-income pool monies that were—he was on notice that—just weren't going to happen, and you came through it very well. We still have challenges in Florida. I hope we can move to Medicaid expansion. But you stayed true to the values and the intent of the Medicaid program, so thank you very much.

I would like to ask about the agency's proposed rule for Medicaid managed care organizations that were issued earlier this year. Given the growing number of Medicaid beneficiaries who receive care through managed care arrangements, it is crucial that we strengthen Federal oversight of these programs to ensure that Federal dollars are being spent wisely. This has my attention especially because a Federal Court Judge in Florida found that Florida's Medicaid program was in violation of Federal law because of low reimbursement rates, failure to provide prompt service and adequate service, failure to provide outreach services as required by the law. Then you had a Supreme Court Decision involving the State of Idaho that said that you can't—private providers cannot challenge low reimbursement rates. So that puts the impetus on HHS to follow through with oversight.

Ms. Yocom, GAO has issued a number of recommendations to CMS to improve Federal oversight of the managed care rate setting process, is that correct? And why does this feel—why does GAO feel that this is necessary?

Ms. YOCOM. Well, it goes back in part to transparency issues, understanding where the money is going and for what purposes. We also did do work just recently that spoke to the fact that neither the Federal Government nor the States in our sample were actually conducting audits of Medicaid managed care organizations, and we recommended that that be changed, that CMS require States to conduct audits both to and by managed care organizations.

Ms. CASTOR. And Ms. Wachino, do you agree?

Ms. WACHINO. I think GAO's concerns helped us really inform some of our thinking about our proposed rule. Ensuring accountability in managed care is vitally important to us because it is where most of our beneficiaries get their care. Medicaid is no longer a fee-for-service program, and managed care has great potential to offer care coordination and meet the needs of low-income Americans, but we really want it to be as strong as possible.

So, to Ms. Yocom's point, part of the proposed rule does include greater auditing by Medicaid managed care plans. We have also proposed new rules with respect to provider enrollment to ensure that providers go through the same screening process when they enroll in a Medicaid managed care plan that they do in a fee-for-service program. And we are making substantial advances in the soundness of the rates that States pay plans.

Ms. CASTOR. Yes. For example, the Federal—I will—I am going to submit these further questions into writing, Mr. Chairman, and I would also like to thank Chairman Emeritus Barton for raising the issue of the Ace Kids Act, and we will look forward to working with CMS on a medical home for children with complex conditions. Thank you very much. I——

Mr. PITTS. The Chair thanks the gentlelady, and now recognizes the gentleman from Kentucky, Mr. Whitfield, 5 minutes for questions.

Mr. WHITFIELD. Thank you very much, and thank the four of you for joining us today, and we appreciate your responsibilities and involvement in the healthcare delivery system in America. As you know, or maybe you don't know, there are about 67 different programs in the Federal Government relating to climate change. And whenever—EPA has been particularly active in that area, and on their regulations they talk about some of the primary benefits relate to health care. Asthma conditions, premature deaths, whatever. And we know that Medicare, 500 billion a year, Medicaid, 330 billion a year, community health centers, around 5 billion a year, I don't know what the cost of Tricare is, but it is primarily about access to health care, which is vitally important.

But one area that I have been reading more and more about recently that disturbs me a great deal relates to antibiotic resistant bacteria. And it is turning out that it is a more significant issue not only nationally, but internationally. And I read an article recently that last year alone in America there were 37,000 deaths relating to infections that could not be treated by antibiotics. And some of the experts are saying that that figure is much lower than reality because the identification system is not sophisticated enough to determine when someone has died because of the bacteria being resistant to antibiotics.

And I have been told that 44—that hospitals in 44 States have had outbreaks of bacteria resistant to antibiotics. Even NIH, our premier research and development institute, has had deaths because of this issue. And I would like to know—you all are involved in the very core of CMS, and HHS, and CDC. Are you aware of some specific programs that are trying to address this problem that faces the American people today?

Ms. WACHINO. Congressman Whitfield, thanks for raising the concerns. I think that HHS shares your concern about making sure that people remain healthy. I would like to go back and consult with my colleagues, particularly in CDC, and get back to you for the record about what they are doing, because I think when it comes to things like surveillance, that is really a primary responsibility of theirs, with Medicaid coverage supporting people, when they unexpectedly fall ill, to make sure they get the services——

Mr. WHITFIELD. But you—well, I appreciate that, because I tell you, I do get upset about it, because we see a plethora of executive orders and regulations relating to asthma, and other things like that, but I am not aware of one executive order or regulation to address this issue, and this is an issue that can really destroy a lot of people in this country and around the world. And the experts that I have heard from, the hospitals that I have talked to, and others, say that this is an epidemic that can be quite serious not only for America, but for the world.

Ms. WACHINO. Thank you for the concern. I am happy to go back and consult with our experts and circle back with you to provide you more information with how we are approaching it.

Mr. PITTS. The Chair thanks the gentleman, now recognize the gentlelady from California, Ms. Matsui, 5 minutes for questions.

Ms. MATSUI. Thank you, Mr. Chairman. As we know, California is the forefront of innovation of many areas, not the least of which is health care. California was an early implementer of Medicaid expansion, and the first State to implement the delivery system reform incentive payment. As we know, Medicaid is a State/Federal partnership, and the ability for the State to implement pieces of the program as it sees fit within Federal guidelines is essential to its success. Of course, the main way that States are able to exercise this flexibility is through the waiver process.

Now, just 2 weeks ago California was the first State to be approved for a 5-year renewal of a different waiver, for specialty mental health services. Previously these types of waivers were only allowed to be renewed in 2-year intervals, but the ACA changed that to allow for 5-year renewals. This is a huge step forward for the nearly one in six California adults, and one in 13 California children with mental health needs.

I am also so pleased that California is also moving forward to apply for new community behavioral health funding in the Medicaid program, which will be available in the form of demonstration projects based on the Excellence in Mental Health Act that I co-authored with my colleague on this committee, Representative Leonard Lance. This demonstration will support California's efforts to integrate mental and physical health. This is so important, as we all know that the head is connected to the body, and we need to treat it that way.

Ms. Wachino, how is a Medicaid program, especially through waivers and demonstration projects, making a difference in the mental health system?

Ms. WACHINO. Thank you for the question. We are working actively on supporting mental health services in a number of areas, and thank you for mentioning the community mental health services program that we released the planning grant announcement for just a few months ago. We were very happy to have that legislation. As you well know, it allows us to pilot approaches in partnership with health centers to advance community-based mental health care, and we are very much looking forward to seeing States apply for those grants. We have had a high interest level so far, and we will look forward to continue working with them.

I think, in addition to that, we have a number of initiatives underway, and a very strong interest level from States in moving towards greater physical and behavioral health integration, and clearly community-based mental health care is a key part of that, and we will be working actively with California, and with other States, to ensure appropriate provision of community-based care.

Ms. MATSUI. Well, thank you. Now, Ms. Wachino, under your leadership CMS recently released the first major proposed update to Medicaid and CHIP managed care rules since 2003, and one of the provisions of the proposed rule would provide flexibility for Medicaid managed care on the so-called IMD exclusion, which prevents Medicaid from paying for inpatient mental health services and facilities with more than 16 beds. Can you please elaborate on that policy, and how it is intended to strike the right balance between the ability to provide inpatient services and emphasis on community-based care?

Ms. WACHINO. Thank you for the question. We have spent a lot of time thinking, and I know many members of Congress have as well, about how to ensure access to mental health services, particularly community mental health services, and we have become aware of a growing need for access to mental health services.

However, we are also trying to approach it cautiously and are very aware of the risk that if we move too far forward, and too fast in moving forward, in terms of allowing Medicaid funding for services to adults in institutions of mental disease—which, as you know, Congresswoman Matsui, is prohibited by statute—that we would risk undermining the progress we have made in serving Medicaid beneficiaries in communities rather than institutions. So our proposed rule tries to strike the balance by proposing to allow States and plans to cover, as part of their capitation rates, short-term stays in institutions of mental disease.

Ms. MATSUI. OK. Thank you. Dr. Schwartz, during your testimony today you noted the importance of Medicaid on our health system safety net. I was particularly interested in your comment that Medicaid often acts as a wraparound insurance for long-term services and supports, as well as employer sponsored insurance and Medicare. Can you please expand on this wraparound role that you described in 10 seconds?

Dr. SCHWARTZ. Yes. I think the primary way is Medicare does not cover long-term services and supports, although it is the primary source of coverage for medical care for the elderly and disabled. Those services have very few sources of private coverage, and Medicaid plays a key role for those populations. It also provides wraparound services for employer-sponsored coverage, primarily for children with disabilities, who have very high costs, particularly for prescription drugs, that may be beyond what their parents' plans pay for.

Ms. MATSUI. OK. Thank you, and I will submit my other questions.

Mr. PITTS. The Chair thanks the gentlelady. I now recognize the gentleman from Illinois, Mr. Shimkus, 5 minutes for questions.

Mr. SHIMKUS. Thank you, Mr. Chairman, and welcome—we have two competing, as you probably heard, hearings going up and down, so I apologize for missing some of the testimony. But to my friend from Kentucky, we do have 21st century cures. Bill is going to be on the floor. Adapt is part of that. It is going to build on gain. This is on the antibiotic resistance issues, which we hope to get, you know, more drugs into the—or to be able to compete. So I do think there is a legislative response. I think his issue was, you know, where is the Government's response? So—but I just throw that out there for information.

Ms. Wachino, in 2008, Mr. Waxman, Dingell, and Mr. Pallone sent a letter to GAO expressing concerns on CMS' implementation of its own policy on 1115s, and we have talked about these today, demonstrations that they be budget neutral. Years later those concerns are still there. GAO has found billions of dollars in increased costs to the Federal Government as a result of waivers that were not budget neutral, a concern that crosses party lines. Can you please explain CMS' process for assessing the budget neutrality of waivers, and how the CMS actuaries are involved in this process?

Ms. WACHINO. Sure. Our approach to budget neutrality, which, as you know, is designed to ensure that costs with the waiver are not higher——

Mr. SHIMKUS. Well, the States have been making promises that they are going to have this new ramped up program that is actually going to be a savings, and we are finding out that they are not.

Ms. WACHINO. Yes. As we work with each State, we try to find a solution. As we have worked them, particularly on budget neutrality, we have made our 1115 waiver approval process more transparent. We have improved our monitoring and evaluation. And particularly with respect to transparency, we put all of our approval documents on medicaid.gov. We also, as you probably know, developed a template for waiver applications that includes a structure for budget neutrality reporting, and we have worked to be consistent in our approaches to budget neutrality across States.

Mr. SHIMKUS. Wouldn't it be prudent to have you all and your actuaries sign off on each demonstration to ensure that it is budget neutral?

Ms. WACHINO. I think we have worked hard to ensure consistency in budget neutrality, and will continue to work hard.

Mr. SHIMKUS. So that brings me to H.R. 2119, which is the bill I dropped, just to really say sign off on it. Have your actuaries actually sign on the dotted line, and put their reputation on the line that, based upon the analysis they have in front of them, that this is going to be—right now, yes, you could put all this stuff out there, but it is not a strong enough signal to say—because we—it is been proven it has not been working. I mean, we are just spending more than what the projected savings would be on the program.

Let me go to one last issue, which I do have time for. If the staff would put the chart up?

FY2014 TOTAL SPENDING $3.5 TRILLION

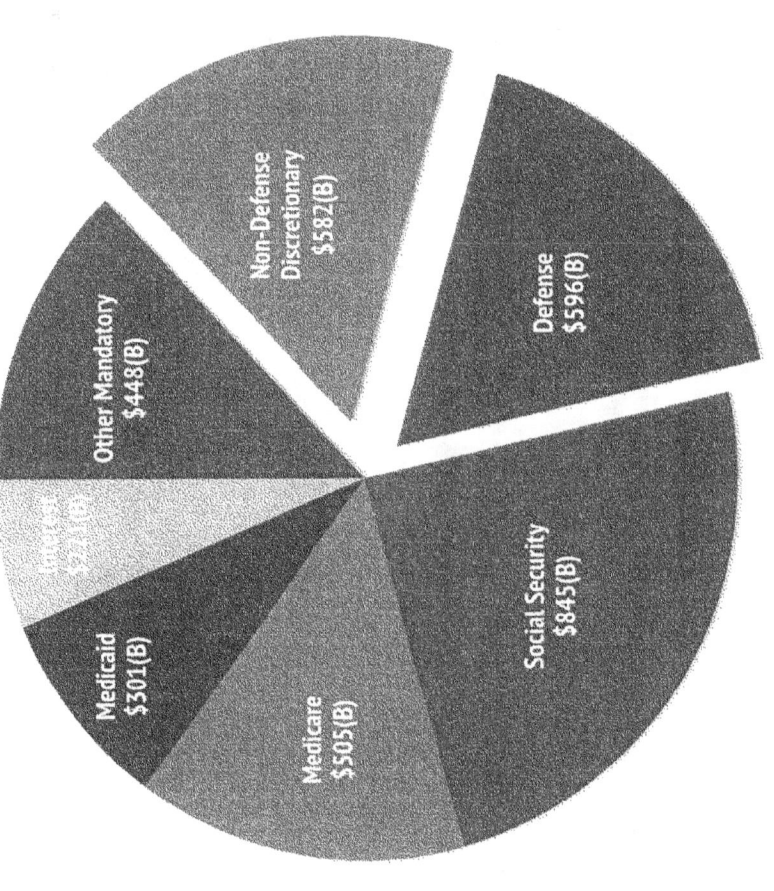

Source: CBO

Mr. SHIMKUS. I talk about this all the time. CBO recently issued a 2015 long-term budget outlook, and has noted that, in a little more than a decade, all the Federal budget will be consumed with entitlements and service on the debt. With respect to Medicaid it said many State Governments will respond to growing costs for Medicaid by restraining payment rates to providers and managed care plans, limiting the services that they choose to cover, or tightening eligibility for those programs so that it serves fewer beneficiaries than it would have otherwise.

This reaffirms a long-term concern of mine that our biggest threat to access to care for our Nation's most vulnerable is the budgetary pressures that States and the Federal Government face in financing our entitlement programs. Yet, in your testimony today, you did not mention the fiscal sustainability of the program at all. Aren't you concerned that unless we make changes our fiscal situation will put beneficiaries' access to care at risk, or do you agree with—disagree with CBO's warnings?

Ms. WACHINO. We are very committed to being strong fiscal stewards of the Medicaid program. I think Medicaid has proven to be a very cost-efficient program. As you saw in some of my colleagues' testimony——

Mr. SHIMKUS. But the point is this, here—that is our budget.

Ms. WACHINO. Um-hum.

Mr. SHIMKUS. The red is mandatory spending. One of those is Medicaid. And the CBO says it is going to grow, so it is going to keep shrinking the blue, which is the discretionary budget, which is all these other things we do, NIH, and all these other things. The CBO report also says that States—and we have seen this. This is not new. States, when they are in budgetary pressure, they start restricting access to Medicaid. Isn't that a threat that you ought to be mentioning when we are doing this let us talk about Medicaid hearing?

Ms. WACHINO. Congressman, we work, again, actively to ensure the sustainability of the program so that it——

Mr. SHIMKUS. So what proposals are you going to provide to us to make this program sustainable?

Ms. WACHINO. Congressman, in the President's budget we proposed proposals around changing the drug rebate——

Mr. SHIMKUS. And that is not in your testimony.

Ms. WACHINO. That is right. My testimony did not address every proposal in the President's budget, but I think it is important to note for the record that there are proposals with respect to changes for durable medical equipment, and to spending for prescription drugs. And we think approaches like that, together with our approaches to strengthening delivery system reforms, are the ways to ensure the sustainability of the program for the future.

Mr. SHIMKUS. Thank you, Mr. Chairman. I will just say actuary changes in entitlement programs. You have to make actuary changes, not nibbling around the edges. And I will yield back my time.

Mr. PITTS. The Chair thanks the gentleman, and now recognize the gentleman from New Mexico, Mr. Luján, 5 minutes for questions.

Mr. Luján. Thank you very much, Mr. Chairman. Ms. Wachino, as you are aware, I have had conversations with you and with Secretary Burwell about concerns with the behavioral health system in New Mexico. At the moment is CMS concerned that New Mexicans enrolled in Medicaid have adequate access to behavioral health services?

Ms. Wachino. Congressman, thank you for working with us and for your continued interest in this issue, and you know that we share concerns about ensuring appropriate access to behavioral health services in New Mexico. We have worked very closely with all States, including New Mexico, to ensure appropriate access to behavioral health care. Specifically, with respect to New Mexico, as you and I have discussed previously, we are working with the State to develop a comprehensive plan to continue and to ensure access. The State has provided us data, which we are reviewing now, and we hope to be able to report out on it soon.

Mr. Luján. So, Ms. Wachino, in 2013 CMS asked the State of New Mexico for a network development plan. Is that the plan you are referring to?

Ms. Wachino. We asked them for a plan. We have actually taken a step back and asked them to go a little bit further than that, and to go review their past plans and their future plans, and provide to us a plan that provides us an assurance that there will be adequate access to mental health services throughout the State.

Mr. Luján. So in 2014 you followed up with a request letter, the same one that you submitted in 2013 to the State of New Mexico, reminding them—it says, we remind the State to submit a network development plan. Has that plan been submitted to CMS?

Ms. Wachino. I will have to go back and check, and I could submit that for the record. I can tell you, Congressman, that we met with the State as recently as June to talk about the need to continue progress forward in this effort. We still have some additional information we are awaiting for the State, and we continue to work with them actively, and look forward to having more to report to you soon.

Mr. Luján. So I appreciate very much that CMS shares concerns. It is also stated in your 2013 letter that CMS continues to be concerned about the transition of behavioral health providers and centennial care. In 2014 the State again worked with the State of New Mexico to ask for some data to be released associated with behavioral health stakeholders.

And there was a letter that was sent to the State of New Mexico in which the State of New Mexico's behavioral health responded to CMS, September 23, 2014. In the letter it says, "As we discussed in our meeting with CMS"—and I am quoting —"and the BHS stakeholders, HSD is anxious to share BH utilization data with the public, but we need to be sure that the data we report is accurate. We are close to confirming the utilization data, and within the next few weeks we expect to release BH utilization data for the first two quarters of centennial care. We understand the importance of data transparency." So it said within the next few weeks. Again, this letter was written September 23.

In an article in the Albuquerque Journal, which is a local paper, published September 24, which is the next morning, at 12:02

a.m.—and I know the press is good, but they can't write an article in a minute, so it probably was written the day before—the spokesperson for HSD says that the data will be presented to the Legislative Finance Committee today. Was someone not being honest with CMS when they sent this letter to you on September 23?

Ms. WACHINO. Congressman, we continue to work as closely as we can with the State to ensure adequate access to behavioral health services. I can go back with my staff and review what the State submitted, and report back to you.

Mr. LUJÁN. Ms. Wachino, has CMS been receiving adequate data yet?

Ms. WACHINO. We have a variety of data sources from the State. We are comparing them to each other, and trying to identify trends and issues with respect to access to behavioral health care.

Mr. LUJÁN. Did CMS receive the data that was publicly reported in the Albuquerque Journal, that was also shared with the New Mexico Legislative Finance Committee on September 24 of 2014? Has CMS received that data?

Ms. WACHINO. Congressman Luján, I know that we have received data, including data that is reported to the legislature from the State. As you know, many of the developments that you have just informed me of precede my tenure at CMCS, so, if I could, I would like to go back and examine the record with my staff who have been working on this.

Mr. LUJÁN. And, Ms. Wachino, with all due respect, these issues were brought up with the meeting with the delegation 6 weeks ago. This is—these are not new questions. The reason I am asking them in this hearing today is because we have not received any answers, and it is frustrating. Especially when it seems that the paper has more access to data than the delegation and CMS does, at least than what is—reporting to us. The way that this information came out was through a FOIA request through a local network of individuals that were concerned in New Mexico. Do—does—do members of Congress have to seek Freedom of Information Act requests to Federal agencies to get data?

Ms. WACHINO. Congressman, as we have committed to you, we would—we are obtaining data from the State, and we have agreed to make it transparent for everyone. And let me say again, we met with the State as recently as early June to try to ensure continued progress in this area, and we are going to continue to work with them and with you to ensure appropriate provision of behavioral health services in the State.

Mr. LUJÁN. All right. Mr. Chairman, I—as you can see, there is some frustration from the delegation in the State of New Mexico in this issue, and it is one that we hope that we can continue to work with the staff and everyone that—from CMS that has been working with us recently. But we need to get these answers to questions that have been asked, and to try to get to the bottom of what is going on.

And I certainly hope that you can share with us. I will submit into the record more questions, Mr. Chairman. A deadline that has been established for when this report were—in 2013—2014. It is now 2015. When is a deadline going to be estab- lished to get this report in? So I thank you, Mr. Chairman, for your indulgence, and I yield back.

Mr. PITTS. The Chair thanks the gentleman, and now recognizes the gentleman from Pennsylvania, Dr. Murphy, 5 minutes for questions.

Mr. MURPHY. Thank you, and good morning. I am going to follow up on some of the questions my colleagues and friends have asked from New Mexico and California, the behavioral thing. I know the GAO report said that behavioral health is a serious problem.

Ms. Wachino, you made reference to the word progress. What progress is being made on the IMD exclusion issue?

Ms. WACHINO. We have been looking very carefully at this issue from the standpoint of wanting to ensure that there is appropriate access to inpatient mental health services and at the same time trying to arrive at an approach that doesn't undermine the progress that we have made——

Mr. MURPHY. That is what I am asking——

Ms. WACHINO [continuing]. Supporting people in the——

Mr. MURPHY [continuing]. What you mean by progress——

Ms. WACHINO [continuing]. Communities.

Mr. MURPHY [continuing]. Is what——

Ms. WACHINO. The most tangible sign of progress is in our proposed managed care rule, where we have proposed to give States the flexibility, and plans the flexibility, to cover, through their capitation rates, short-term stays in their——

Mr. MURPHY. "Short-term" meaning?

Ms. WACHINO. "Short-term" meaning—I think the standard is up to 15 days. I can tell you that we reviewed preliminary data from the Medicaid emergency psychiatric demonstration, which I know you are familiar with, and use that to base the standard for the short-term stay.

Mr. MURPHY. Some things about that have been—I am concerned that a short-term stay of 15 days is insufficient, because it may take a couple weeks to get off of one medication, couple weeks to get back on another one. But we don't—but that is different from residential care. I am looking at things that I think are valuable at a less than 30 days average rate.

But when you are looking at these issues, and helping States do that, are you looking at other dependent variables, such as suicide rates, drug overdose rates, arrests, incarcerations, homelessness, ER boarding costs, are any of those things you are looking at?

Ms. WACHINO. I think, Congressman, your question points to—at the end of the day we should be looking at health outcomes.

Mr. MURPHY. Um-hum.

Ms. WACHINO. When we fund Medicaid services, I believe that the evaluation of the Medicaid emergency psychiatric demonstration will inform our policy in this area significantly. We don't have evaluation results yet.

Mr. MURPHY. And I just want to make sure, as you are pursuing that—and this is what I want to find out, what your dependent variables are in your study. A recent report that was just—I just read from the Arkansas legislature, might want to look that up. It looked at States like Oregon, Georgia, Texas, and found that the rates—the cost of incarcerating someone with mental illness could be 10 times higher than the rate of serving them in the community.

Obviously this would be a huge issue, especially if you have the revolving door of people in and out of jails, show up in emergency rooms, back in the community, we are not serving anybody well that way. I am sure you would agree. That is heartless, and that is— we don't do that in this country. Unfortunately, we do that, but it is a serious concern.

But with regard to that, I also want to talk about legislation I have that this committee has been dealing with my legislation, Helping Families in Mental Health Crisis Act. We are trying to reform the whole system. And one of the ways that we look at this is to help—is through promoting stronger enforcement of mental health parity. And recently CMS proposed a rulemaking that would apply purely to beneficiaries served by Medicaid and managed care, which have far reaching positive implications, if complied with.

On another area, though, I have strong concerns about the proposed rule's exclusion of long-term care services from MHPAEA, parity protections. Long-term care services, inpatient and community based, are critical to many individuals with mental health and substance abuse disorders, particularly the medicated CHIP population. And CMS has clear authority and statutory obligation to apply parity to all covered benefits under these programs, yet the proposed rule doesn't even define long-term care services, or identify the types of services that apply. Can you address this flaw in the proposed rule with regard to the definition of that?

Ms. WACHINO. As you know, the comment period on our proposed mental health parity rule, which we think is a very substantial advance in coverage of mental health services in the Medicaid program, just recently closed. We are reviewing the comments now, and I would fully expect that the question of whether these protections also extend to long-term services is something that we will receive a lot of comments on, and that we will actively consider as we finalize the rule.

Mr. MURPHY. Thank you. I hope—what is important to all these rules, in looking at behavioral health, is when—you also talk about progress in this issue is—I think we are also—so all—you have the IMD exclusion. A lot of people can't get care for the crisis, period. We don't want people—we don't ever want to bring back the asylums, but we want people to have an option for crisis, instead of being boarded in an emergency room. We have had testimony in my Oversight Committee that boarding would take place for hours, days, weeks, and months. Terrible place for a person to be strapped to a gurney as these things go on.

But part of the concern also is that there are just simply not enough providers. Not enough psychiatrists, not enough clinical psychologists, not enough clinical social workers, who deal with the severely mentally ill. And so I am hoping that is also something you are looking at as well. It has an impact upon the reimbursement and—provision of these. As you are looking at working out these partnerships with States, we have to have ways of getting more people out there, because nothing is worse than telling someone, there is just no room for you, and there is no one to see you. I yield back.

Mr. PITTS. The Chair thanks the gentleman. I now recognize the gentleman from Oregon, Mr. Schrader, 5 minutes for questions.

Mr. SCHRADER. Thank you, Mr. Chairman, I appreciate it. Ms. Wachino, could you comment a little bit on Medicaid spending per beneficiary compared to private insurance over this past decade?

Ms. WACHINO. Sure. Thank you for the question. When you look at per capita—per beneficiary costs, Medicaid costs have been recently growing more slowly than the per beneficiary costs in private insurance. And I believe I saw in my colleague's testimony projections that, on a per beneficiary basis, Medicaid costs are expected to grow more slowly than private insurance. Of course, we are putting a number of tools in place focused on delivery system reform to ensure that we continue to do the best possible job of maintaining Medicaid's cost efficiency.

Mr. SCHRADER. CBO would apparently agree with you on that. Ms. Yocom, just a quick comment. I—as we celebrate the 50th anniversary of Medicaid, the program is changing. We are moving past the old fee-for-service—pay for, you know a widget or a particular service—and going to this managed care type of model, where we are treating the whole patient a little bit, I think to answer Dr. Murphy's concerns, and others. Is GAO prepared to audit outcome-based results versus just how the money is spent?

I mean, in our last hearing Ms. Iritani and others in GAO talking about how the money is spent. And certainly when you are just monitoring, you know, individual dollars going out, that is appropriate. But, as a policymaker of the 21st century, I would rather monitor outcomes. I am not sure I can evaluate the appropriateness of an expenditure, but I can evaluate whether or not we are getting results. Is GAO prepared to work along those lines?

Ms. YOCOM. We would be glad to work with you on putting together work in that area. We have also done some work looking at managed care utilization rates, and did find a wide variety of utilization rates across the 19 States that we looked at. And some of this did appear to be related to whether or not a beneficiary was enrolled in Medicaid for the full year versus a partial year.

Mr. SCHRADER. All right. That will be fun to work with you on. I know my own State, much like I guess Kentucky, the Medicaid expansion—what was occurring before this was going on, before the ACA, and with the ACA, last year and a half we added 400,000 people to the Medicaid rolls. Big active outreach by folks in our State. We also have 25 percent of our population on Medicaid. It is not a—at least they have access—that great a portion of the population, I think.

Ms. Wachino, pleased to see you reference Oregon's program in your testimony. It is a fairly innovative outcome-based approach, where we are trying to keep costs down. Actually, half of the projected rate for Medicaid growth nationally, from 4 percent down to 2 percent, in the same time get better outcomes.

I commented last year about results from a year ago, and I guess just recently new data came out, with emergency room visits down 22 percent amongst these coordinate care organizations that deal with mental health, hopefully dental health, as well as the fiscal health of the people. Short-term complications from diabetes down 27 percent with this coordinated care approach. Hospital admissions from COPD, chronic obstructive pulmonary disease, down 60 percent. You know, and that is one of the long-term cost drivers,

81

unfortunately, of a lot of health care in this country, whether you are on Medicaid, Medicare, or private insurance. Can you comment a little bit on what CMS may be learning from what you are seeing in Oregon, and how you might evaluate future waivers from different States?

Ms. WACHINO. Sure. I think we will be looking very carefully at the results of the Oregon demonstration. And I am not yet familiar with the results you just shared, so thank you for that, and improving the population health. Oregon Committed is part of the 1115 waiver to very robust cost quality goals. And as we review the success of the waiver with them and of their coordinated care in serving Medicaid beneficiaries, we will want to look at cost, and quality, and how it is achieving those goals.

Mr. SCHRADER. Good, good. Well, I think it is the future of medicine. Frankly, the future of Federal budgeting in general, rather than trying to dictate to different agencies or different providers around the country how to do things. Let us talk with them, share concerns about outcomes and where we are trying to go, monitor those and spend money there, hopefully a little more efficiently. With that I yield back. Thank you, Mr. Chairman.

Mr. PITTS. The Chair thanks the gentleman. I now recognize the gentleman from New Jersey, Mr. Lance, 5 minutes for questions.

Mr. LANCE. Thank you very much, and good morning to you all. And I apologize for shuttling between two subcommittees. I think this is a very interesting hearing, and I want to learn more about Medicaid.

To Ms. Wachino, when the program began 50 years ago, I assume that greater expenditures were in Medicare than Medicaid, is that accurate, 50 years ago?

Ms. WACHINO. Congressman, I would have to go back and look at the history——

Mr. LANCE. Well——

Ms. WACHINO [continuing]. To——

Mr. LANCE. Well, perhaps someone else on the panel. I presume at some point the line crossed, and the greater expenditure was on Medicaid than Medicare. Can anybody on the panel enlighten me on that?

Ms. YOCOM. I know that—and I attended a conference a couple of years ago where it was mentioned that combined Federal and State spending on Medicaid had just exceeded that of Medicare, total Medicare spending, and that would have been maybe a year or two ago.

Mr. LANCE. Combined Federal/State on Medicaid?

Ms. YOCOM. Correct.

Mr. LANCE. Whereas Medicare, of course, is primarily a Federal program. I wonder whether this was anticipated. The figures I have is that 70 million people utilize Medicaid, is that right, in this country? We have 310, 315 million people? Is that right? Seventy million people?

Ms. YOCOM. Yes.

Mr. LANCE. And has that increased because of the terrible recession? I know it increased as well because of the ACA. I am familiar with that, and the fact that some States have expanded Medicaid, and others have not, and that is a great debate in this country.

And New Jersey is one of those States with a Republican Governor that expanded Medicaid. But do you think that the numbers have increased as well due to the fact that we are not in as robust economic times as we all would like?

Ms. YOCOM. We have done work looking at the effects during the economic downturns, and Medicaid enrollment does go up during an economic downturn. It also recovers—it is related to unemployment, of course——

Mr. LANCE. Yes.

Ms. YOCOM [continuing]. And unemployment, it tends to be a lagging indicator, so the recovery is also slower. And so you tend to get people on Medicaid more quickly, and they stay longer.

Mr. LANCE. Now, the unemployment rate is whatever it is, 5.3 percent. It is lower than it was. Is there a correlation as well with the labor participation rate?

Ms. YOCOM. Yes, there is.

Mr. LANCE. Um-hum.

Ms. YOCOM. Yes.

Mr. LANCE. Yes. I mean, people cite the lower unemployment rate. I think that is half the picture. There is also a dramatically lower labor participation rate in this country. So there would be a correlation between Medicaid and the labor participation rate?

Ms. YOCOM. Right. Our work relied on the employment-to-population ratio.

Mr. LANCE. Um-hum. And that is significantly lower than it has been in the last 50 years. Would that be an accurate statement?

Ms. YOCOM. I couldn't answer that.

Mr. LANCE. I think it is the lowest it has been since at least 1980, something like that. Thank you. Well, I want to learn more about this, because it is such an important part of the public policy of this country for the last 50 years.

To CMS in particular, and this is a long and complicated question, and has lots of jargon in it, CMS has indicated the oversight of a program the size and scope of Medicaid requires robust, timely, and accurate data to ensure efficient financial and program performance, support policy analysis and ongoing improvement, identify potential fraud, waste, and abuse, and enable data driver decision making.

Work conducted by the OIG in 2013 raised questions about the completeness and accuracy of the Transformed Medicaid Statistical Information System, TMSIS, data upon national implementation. CMS has since stated its goal of having all States submitting data in the TMSIS file format by 2015. Could you please describe the actions you are taking to ensure that this occurs?

Ms. WACHINO. Sure. If it helps with the jargon, Congressman, we call it TMSIS, and it is a data——

Mr. LANCE. TMSIS?

Ms. WACHINO. TMSIS.

Mr. LANCE. I have learned something this morning.

Ms. WACHINO. And it is CMS' investment in getting stronger, better, more comprehensive, and faster data, and how our program is working.

Mr. LANCE. Um-hum.

83

Ms. WACHINO. We have made substantial advances in TMSIS implementation this year. Our first State started submitting data in May, and we expect to have nearly all States submitting data by the end of the year. So we are moving forward and very eager to start sharing the data with external stakeholders for analysis, and using it for our own program management.

Mr. LANCE. Thank you. My time has expired, and I look forward to working with all of you.

Mrs. ELLMERS [presiding]. The Chair now recognizes Mr. Sarbanes from Maryland for 5 minutes.

Mr. SARBANES. Thank you, Madam Chair. Thank you all for your testimony. I am very interested in the money following the person initiative, and I wanted to hear a little bit more about that. When I was in private practice as a healthcare attorney, I had the opportunity, in Maryland, to work on a program where Medicaid—the Medicaid program assigned a certain number of slots where assisted living facilities could qualify for Medicaid reimbursement, which doesn't typically happen when you have skilled nursing care, which is covered, but doesn't extend into the assisted living arena.

But the observation was there were sort of people in that inner section who could actually be treated in assisted living facilities, as opposed to going into skilled nursing, and could—that could be done at much less cost, and so why not try and explore that opportunity, potentially broaden it. And if we can continue to design that expansion or initiative going forward, it could produce tremendous savings, as well as being better for patients. And that can include exploring what sorts of treatments or reimbursement can occur in the home, right? So you are not even getting into institutional care of any kind.

So I was just curious, what is the status of exploring this—what I consider a new frontier, particularly as the demographics of the wave of our seniors is coming at us full force?

Ms. WACHINO. Congressman, thank you for the question. We have spent a lot of time at CMS moving towards approaches that promote care—the most community-based care possible. And there is, as you note, a spectrum of different types of providers that can serve those individuals. Money Follows The Person is one vehicle by which we have worked with States towards that goal. We also have worked with them through the balancing incentive programs, and through their home and community-based service waivers.

Currently, we have been assessing some of the things we have learned from our work with States through Money Follows The Person, and similar programs, and using it to inform our efforts with all States moving towards greater community integration, and would be happy to follow up with you on some of the particular things we have learned, and in particular the interaction with assisted living facilities.

Mr. SARBANES. Are you—I mean, are you seeing some real potential savings opportunities there?

Ms. WACHINO. I would like to look back more carefully at the fiscal impacts. I can say with certainty that we are seeing high rates of satisfaction from our beneficiaries as they move forward with greater community care. So we will circle back with you and provide evidence and impact on the cost.

Mr. SARBANES. I would love to get more information about that, and maybe collaborate with you——

Ms. WACHINO. We will follow up——

Mr. SARBANES [continuing]. Going forward.

Ms. WACHINO [continuing]. With you. Thank you for the question.

Mr. SARBANES. Thank you very much. I yield back my time.

Mrs. ELLMERS. The gentleman yields back. The Chair now recognizes Mr. Bilirakis from Florida for 5 minutes.

Mr. BILIRAKIS. Thank you, Madam Chair. I appreciate you very much, and I want to thank you for your testimony.

Ms. Yocom, in your statement you—for—to your report titled Medicaid Demonstrations, Approval Criteria and Documentation Needs To Show How Spending Furthers Medicaid Objectives, you highlight how HHS has approved questionable methods and assumptions for spending estimates without providing adequate documentation. You also mentioned HHS does not have explicit criteria explaining how it determines how spending in the demonstration program furthers Medicaid objectives.

You also note their approval documents are not always clear on what expenditures are for, and how it will promote Medicaid objections—objectives. Can you talk about what recommendations have GAO made in this area that have not been accepted or implemented by HHS or CMS?

Ms. IRITANI. I will answer that question. Yes, we have made several recommendations to CMS around those issues that you point out. One is to issue criteria regarding how CMS assesses whether or not approved new spending under demonstrations will further objectives. A second is to apply that criteria in the documentation and make the documentation transparent. And a third relates to providing assurances in the documentation that approved spending will not duplicate other Federal funding sources. CMS agreed with the latter two and partially agreed with our recommendation to issue criteria on how they assess spending.

Mr. BILIRAKIS. Have these recommendations been implemented, and then why not, Ms. Wachino?

Ms. WACHINO. We have implemented the GAO's recommendations with respect to ensuring our approval documents are clear with respect to the criteria we use, with ensuring that there is no duplication of Federal fundings, and ensuring that we are consistently and clearly articulating when we determine that a particular authority meets the objectives of the Medicaid program.

We moved forward with that implementation, with implementing those policies while the report was still in draft, and so have worked very actively over the past several months to ensure that our approval documents are clear.

Mr. BILIRAKIS. Ms. Yocom, what do you have to say about that? Do you agree?

Ms. YOCOM. I really have to defer to Ms. Iritani. She is the expert in this area from GAO.

Mr. BILIRAKIS. Please.

Ms. IRITANI. We have not reviewed the changes that Ms. Wachino has said that they have made, so we would need to do that in order to see how they are documenting their approvals.

That said we still feel strongly that there should be more transparent criteria for how they assess whether or not new spending
will further Medicaid objectives.

Mr. BILIRAKIS. OK. Please get back to our committee after a review of these objectives, OK? Please. I am sure most of the committee is interested in this, not all.

Ms. Wachino, you probably know about Puerto Rico's financial
challengers, which are rather severe, I am sure you will agree. A
recent morning consult story highlighted the contrast in treatment
that Puerto Rico receives under Federal healthcare programs. For
example, Puerto Rico has a rather low spending cap on its program. Are you monitoring the rate at which Puerto Rico is spending its Medicaid funds, and do you worry it will exhaust those
funds well before 2019?

Ms. WACHINO. We are looking very closely at the overall situation in Puerto Rico, including its Medicaid spending, very aware
that there are a bunch of very strong concerns about the finances
of Puerto Rico, and considering what approaches we might take.
Last year, in approving some of their benefits, we offered flexibility, and they took us up on it, and—with respect to their administration, and we are continuing to look at the spending in the program, and options for assisting the Commonwealth.

Mr. BILIRAKIS. In your estimation, will they exhaust the funds
before 2019?

Ms. WACHINO. I would have to go back and look at that, Congressman, but I am happy to submit a response for the record.

Mr. BILIRAKIS. Thank you. Ms. Wachino, CMS proposes to develop the Medicaid managed care quality rate system for managed
care organizations in all States, which would presumably be similar to the Medicare Advantage five-star rating system. However,
research shows that CMS' current start system undervalues care
provided to beneficiaries with low socioeconomic status. This is an
area of growing bipartisan concern. So how does CMS plan to address this issue, especially since all the Medicaid beneficiaries are
presumably low-income?

Ms. WACHINO. Congressman, thank you for the question. Our
proposal to implement the quality rating system is designed to
make sure that low-income people are able to compare quality
across plans and select plans in the same way that individuals in
the private market and in Medicare Advantage can. We think that
is a substantial advance in quality for our program, and an assist
to our consumers.

We do plan on—should we finalize the rule, which, as you know,
is out for public comment now, we propose to have pretty lengthy
implementation schedules, and a very substantial public input
process so that we could identify the strengths of other quality rating systems, bring them to bear in ours, and make any needed adjustments that we need to to account, to your point, for the low-
income nature of our populations, and the fact that our populations
differ in some very important respects from those of Medicare and
commercial insurers.

Mr. BILIRAKIS. OK. Thank you very much, and I yield back,
Madam Chair.

Mrs. ELLMERS. Thank you. The gentleman yields back. The Chair now recognizes the gentleman from California, Mr. Cárdenas, for 5 minutes.

Mr. CÁRDENAS. Thank you very much, Madam Chairwoman. Appreciate the opportunity for us to dialogue with the witnesses. I just wanted to remind all of us that one of the main points of Medicaid was to eventually get to the point where we have protection or security against the economic effects of sickness for all Americans. In addition to that, President Truman, one of his statements included the line that talks about health security for all.

On that note, as a result of the Affordable Care Act, our country currently holds the lowest rate of the uninsured in the history of this Nation. In 2014 alone Medicaid helped reduce the number of uninsured Americans from 43 million to 26 million. Is that about right, Ms. Wachino?

Ms. WACHINO. I do know that we have made really—very substantial advances in reducing the uninsured rate, and it is an accomplishment we are very proud of.

Mr. CÁRDENAS. OK. Well, I would like you to take it back to all of the hard working folks within your department, to let them know how much not only do those 43, down to 26, Americans who now have health care appreciate all of your good hard work, but also at the same time that it is a vision that hopefully we can see in our lifetime, where we could see that 26 million go down to nothing. In addition to that, one of the things that I noticed, as a politician myself, is that many people try to use the word entitlement program as though it is a bad word. But yet, at the same time, I prefer to call it a safety net, which is a good thing, because it brings dignity, and actually saves lives for many Americans, especially hard working poor Americans.

Speaking of the hard working poor, my first question goes to you, Dr. Schwartz. Thank you very much for your testimony today. One of the issues that is very important to my constituents is the availability of health care to all constituents in my district. But my district being 70 percent Latino, a disproportionate representation of uninsured is within the Latino community in my district, and around the country. And this is despite the fact that among these uninsured Latino households, 82 percent of those households are part of a hard working employed family.

So we are not talking about people who choose not to work, we are talking about people who are the working poor, which it— which, in my opinion, is part of the backbone of what makes this country great, people willing to go to work every single day and be able to work for whatever meager means people are willing to pay them, yet at the same time they do it every single day, and then have to worry about whether or not somebody is going to get sick in their family, and if they are going to have a catastrophic change to their entire finances for maybe one or two generations to come. On that note, has MACPAC undertaken any work looking specifi- cally at barriers to enrollment that may still exist in the Latino community?

Dr. SCHWARTZ. No, we haven't. We have done work looking at the experience of different minority communities in accessing services, and I believe Medicaid mirrors much of the rest of the health system in that different minority populations do experience higher barriers to care. And that is an area, as I said in my written statement, that we are interested in the experiences of groups within the Medicaid population, because they are so diverse, and how their different experience of care relate, and what policy solutions might be appropriate, given the different experiences.

Mr. CÁRDENAS. OK. Please keep in mind at all times that it is not just language barriers, cultural as well are some of the barriers out there.

Ms. Wachino, what types of initiatives are underway to help ensure that we reach Latino and other minority communities where individuals may be eligible for coverage, particularly in the wake of Medicaid expansion?

Ms. WACHINO. Thank you for the question. I think we are very interested in making sure that Latino residents across the country get coverage. And, clearly, one way to do that is by taking up Medicaid expansion, as California has. We also are working actively to ensure that eligible Latinos, working families, I mean, the Latino community, enroll in coverage.

And, frequently, that requires outreach and application support, so we work with programs like our navigator programs to make sure that people have support in applying for coverage, provide the information they need to to get an eligibility determination and enroll.

Mr. CÁRDENAS. OK. Thank you. Ms. Wachino, with over 25 million low-income Americans nationwide who are unable to see a primary care physician, I believe telemedicine could provide an incredibly effective way to improve the healthcare system for everyone. Could you expand on the particular benefits for using telemedicine with dual eligibles who are unable to visit their doctor due to illness or immobility? And not just in rural areas, but also in higher populated areas as well.

Ms. WACHINO. We have moved forward with telemedicine in a number of states. It is an approach that a State can take to promote access to care without even seeking a State plan amendment from us. I can look at the particular use of telemedicine for the dual eligible population and circle back with you, and provide information for the record about specifics to that population.

Mr. CÁRDENAS. Thank you very much.

Mrs. ELLMERS. Thank you. The gentleman yields. The Chair now recognizes the gentlelady from Tennessee, Mrs. Blackburn, for 5 minutes.

Mrs. BLACKBURN. Thank you, Madam Chairman, and I am going to make Mr. Pallone's day, because I am going to say TennCare, and talk about TennCare with you all. And I know you are very familiar with it, Ms. Wachino. There is a lot of frustration with that program, but embodied in that in part is frustration that some of the States who have been under the waivers for years, and doing the same thing for decades, have to keep coming back to you every 3 to 5 years for permission once again. So would it not make sense to start to grant the States a longer reprieve, and give them a longer path to certainty or permanence on these issues?

Ms. WACHINO. Thank you for the question, Congresswoman Blackburn. As you know, we work very actively with each State to try to develop——

Mrs. BLACKBURN. This is a yes or no.

Ms. WACHINO [continuing]. For the State. We have been looking very actively, and I think Secretary Burwell spoke with the Governors about this in February, about streamlining our renewal process. It is very important——

Mrs. BLACKBURN. OK, it is a yes or a no question.

Ms. WACHINO. I think that there are ways, and we are working on them now——

Mrs. BLACKBURN. OK.

Ms. WACHINO [continuing]. To——

Mrs. BLACKBURN. Thank you.

Ms. WACHINO [continuing]. Streamline——

Mrs. BLACKBURN. Ms. Yocom——

Ms. WACHINO [continuing]. Renewals.

Mrs. BLACKBURN [continuing]. You want to weigh in on that? No? OK. All right. Well, maybe you want to weigh in on this one. CMS has all these rules—and again, this comes from my guys at the State level—on transparency and required timeframes for the States when they are applying for their waivers, but then CMS doesn't hold themselves to this own standard, and sometimes it can take forever to get an answer from you. So should you not be held to the same standard that you are foisting on the States, to meet deadlines and timelines and to give some certainty?

Ms. WACHINO. Congresswoman, we are very committed to working with States quickly to evaluate waiver requests——

Mrs. BLACKBURN. OK, let us pick up the pace, then.

Ms. WACHINO. May I——

Mrs. BLACKBURN [continuing]. Yocom—no, ma'am. Ms. Yocom, you want to—or Ms. Iritani? Yes. I am just short on time. You can expand in——

Ms. WACHINO. I will.

Mrs. BLACKBURN [continuing]. Form. Thank you. Ms. Iritani?

Ms. IRITANI. Yes, we have heard concerns from States about the lengthy time to get waivers——

Mrs. BLACKBURN. Yes.

Ms. IRITANI [continuing]. Renewed and approved, and we have seen wide variation in approval times. You know, our concern is around the lack of standards and criteria, and we think that those would help bring more transparency——

Mrs. BLACKBURN. So, to be more definitive, lay out a timeline, give the States some certainty, and maybe not make them come back every 3 to 5 years. That makes some sense, doesn't it?

Ms. IRITANI. We believe that there is more need for oversight——

Mrs. BLACKBURN. OK.

Ms. IRITANI [continuing]. So there is the——

Mrs. BLACKBURN. Let me go to a question on enrollment. States are required to enroll applicants who attest to being citizens, or to having legal immigration status, and then are thereby eligible for Medicaid. States receiving Federal matching funding for the care during this reasonable opportunity period. But, as a result, and I am hearing this from some of my State legislators, individuals who are not citizens or eligible permanent residents may be enrolled, and receiving Medicaid. So does CMS think it is appropriate for Federal taxpayer Medicaid dollars to be expended on individuals who are neither citizens nor eligible residents? Ms. Wachino?

Ms. WACHINO. Congresswoman, we think it is very important for us to make accurate eligibility determinations. When people apply for Medicaid coverage, they attest to their citizenship. We verify that electronically through the hub, which is a major advance for us in making accurate eligibility determinations. If someone is not able——

Mrs. BLACKBURN. OK.

Ms. WACHINO [continuing]. To——

Mrs. BLACKBURN. Then let me ask you this. Should we not withhold those benefits until such time as their—certainty and a verification process is completed?

Ms. WACHINO. Congresswoman, the—under the statute, individuals have a reasonable opportunity——

Mrs. BLACKBURN. OK.

Ms. WACHINO [continuing]. Period. They attest to citizenship, and then we, during that period, verify it.

Mrs. BLACKBURN. OK.

Ms. WACHINO. If they are found to be ineligible, they are determined ineligible.

Mrs. BLACKBURN. OK. Let us look at billing privileges. And Obamacare explicitly requires that States suspend the billing privileges of most providers that have been terminated or revoked by another State, or by Medicare. However, more than 5 years after enactment, banned providers are still receiving many of these Medicaid payments. So what steps is CMS taking to ensure, once again, that taxpayer dollars are not going to those that are prohibited, should be prohibited, from receiving this money? And are you taking steps to recoup Federal dollars paid to prohibited providers by State Medicaid programs?

And, in the same vein, how are you dealing—how does CMS deal with companies that have been found guilty of fraud and should not be receiving taxpayer dollars, but they go out and they sell themselves so they can be renamed, and still get taxpayer dollars? I would like to hear from you on this, and, Ms. Yocom, I would also like to—Ms. Yocom, let us start with you, as a matter of fact.

Ms. YOCOM. Certainly. We have done work in this area, and we did identify, in terms of providers, issues where individuals who did have suspended or revoked licenses were receiving payments. We also have identified some providers who are dead who are receiving payments.

Mrs. BLACKBURN. And erroneous payments amounted to how much last year?

Ms. YOCOM. I would have to get back——

Mrs. BLACKBURN. OK.

Ms. YOCOM [continuing]. With you on that. Yes.

Mrs. BLACKBURN. OK.

Ms. YOCOM. Yes.

Mrs. BLACKBURN. OK. Ms. Wachino, you want to comment on that?

Ms. WACHINO. Yes, Congresswoman. It is very important to us that we ensure that the providers serving Medicaid beneficiaries are appropriate, both so that they get the care they need, and so that we are ensuring——

Mrs. BLACKBURN. That is not the question that I have asked you. I have asked you what you are doing about it. So why don't you submit for the committee an answer about what you are doing about erroneous payments, and what you are doing about providers that are not eligible getting this money. I yield back my time.

Mr. GREEN. Madam Chair, can I just have 30 seconds? Ms. Wachino, I understand that under law that—and California is the only State that expanded Medicaid to undocumented children, and—but they don't get the Federal match. Is that true? If it is a State decision?

Ms. WACHINO. I am not familiar with the particular circumstances in California, but Medicaid generally does not provide comprehensive coverage for immigrants. There is a limited provision for emergency care only.

Mr. GREEN. OK. Thank you.

Mrs. ELLMERS. I would just ask that you provide us with the accurate documented material——

Ms. WACHINO. I will happy to do that——

Mrs. ELLMERS [continuing]. To the committee, since this issue has been raised. Thank you.

Ms. WACHINO. I will happy to do that for the record, as well as to respond to——

Mrs. ELLMERS. Thank you.

Ms. WACHINO [continuing]. Ms. Blackburn's question——

Mrs. ELLMERS. Thank you.

Ms. WACHINO [continuing]. About provider enrollment.

Mrs. ELLMERS. Thank you. The Chair now recognizes Mr. Pallone from New Jersey for 5 minutes, the ranking member of our committee.

Mr. PALLONE. Thank you, Madam Chairwoman. I was going to ask unanimous consent to include in the record two new health affair studies that just came out that found evidence that Medicaid expansion has made patients' and hospitals' bottom lines healthier. I think you have copies of them.

Mrs. ELLMERS. We have not had a chance to review that, so I reserve——

Mr. PALLONE. Let me hand them over to you, then, take a look.

Mrs. ELLMERS. We will consider at a later date, before the hearing adjourns.

Mr. PALLONE. OK, thanks. I was going to say to Ms. Blackburn that I hadn't—she left, but that I hadn't heard about TennCare so often that I actually forgot about it, but she brought it up again, but she is not here, so, sorry.

All of our witnesses here today have an important and different perspective to share about Medicaid and its 50th anniversary. I wanted to ask first, Ms. Wachino, as we reflect on Medicaid's 50th year, what do you see as the most significant changes to the program from the standpoint of low-income consumers?

Ms. WACHINO. Well, Medicaid has grown and evolved over time. I think some of the biggest change—we have seen over time its role expand for a variety of populations: coverage of pregnant women to ensure access to strong prenatal care and promote lower rates of infant mortality, expansions to coverage of people with chronic conditions, like HIV.

I think if I had to choose two developments just to single out, the first would be the coverage of low-income children, that I know was led out of this committee, through both Medicaid expansions, and later CHIP, which really built on that. And if you look at the record on the impact of that coverage, it has clearly been a critical support for low-income families through thick economic times and thin.

The second would be the coverage expansion for Medicaid to low-income adults under the Affordable Care Act, which I think really solidifies Medicaid's role as the base for a strong system of health coverage in the United States. And I think, as we work with more States to implement it, we will see that base firmly solidified.

Mr. PALLONE. Thank you. And then, Dr. Schwartz, MACPAC was formed fairly recently, but the Commissioners and MACPAC staff have already proven to be an invaluable resource to both sides of the aisle. What, in your opinion, have been some of Medicaid's greatest advancements?

Dr. SCHWARTZ. I think, to follow up on Ms. Wachino's comments, the program has really transformed over its lifetime from a program that provided medical care to a very small group of low-income families who were receiving cash assistance to a much larger program that takes a much more proactive role in delivery system design, in payment initiatives to improve the delivery of care to a broader set of populations: children, pregnant women, adults, and, of course, people with disabilities.

I think the other is the very significant shift in the delivery of long-term care from institutions into homes and communities, allowing people with disabilities to remain in their homes and active in their communities.

Mr. PALLONE. Thank you. Could I just ask, Ms. Wachino, if you would take—I have just got about a minute and 20 seconds of my time. Could you just talk about CMS' work over the last 5 years on program integrity as a result of the Affordable Care Act tools? Ms. WACHINO. Yes. We take our program responsibilities very seriously.

I participate in them. They are led out of our Center for Program Integrity, but we work in concert. We have worked actively over the last 5 years on a comprehensive Medicaid integrity plan. We have worked to do program integrity reviews of each State, because program integrity in Medicaid is a shared State and Federal effort. We both have responsibilities.

But one of the most tangible things we have done is improve the process of ensuring that high risk providers do not enter into our programs. We have employed and worked with States on high risk provider screening, and we have given States access to the same data to screen out providers that Medicare uses. So I think we have made very substantial advances. I think some of the data you heard about earlier is from 2011, and predates some of our recent accomplishments.

Mr. PALLONE. All right. Thank you very much. Thank you, Madam Chairwoman.

Mrs. ELLMERS. Thank you to the ranking member, and, without objection, the documents that you provided will be submitted into the record.

[The information appears at the conclusion of the hearing.]

Mrs. ELLMERS. The Chair now recognizes myself for 5 minutes. Thank you to our panel for being here. Ms. Wachino, in the most recent actuarial report on the financial outlook for Medicaid, CMS reports that the projected annual growth rate for Medicaid expenditures is faster than the projection of annual GDP growth. The actuary noted that, "should these trends continue as projected under current law, Medicaid's share of both Federal and State budgets would continue to expand, despite any other changes to the program, budget expenditures, or budget revenues."

As a representative from a State that has not expanded Medicaid, in North Carolina, I have two questions. Given that this would crowd out other important fiscal priorities for both State and Federal Government, don't you think that there are changes that need to be made to the program to alter this current trend?

Ms. WACHINO. Congresswoman Ellmers, thank you for the question. We have worked very actively to ensure that the program is on a sound fiscal footing——

Mrs. ELLMERS. Um-hum.

Ms. WACHINO [continuing]. Generally, and, you know, with respect to expansion in particular. I think we have put in common-sense reforms to ensure accountability of funds through——

Mrs. ELLMERS. Um-hum.

Ms. WACHINO [continuing]. Activities like reviewing our rates and ensuring that we are not overpaying for services. I think, in addition to that, you see from the administration proposals like changes to the drug rebate that are designed to ensure that some of the major cost drivers in our program are addressed. So I think we can work, and we do work, and we look forward to working with you for really——

Mrs. ELLMERS. Um-hum.

Ms. WACHINO [continuing]. Putting the program on a sound fiscal footing.

Mrs. ELLMERS. Well, thank you for that. I would like to ask, have these changes, or proposed changes, resulted in any decreases in spending up to this point?

Ms. WACHINO. We do know in some States that have embarked on delivery system reform that there have been reductions in things like hospitalizations——

Mrs. ELLMERS. Um-hum.

Ms. WACHINO [continuing]. That have resulted in cost savings. There are a couple of——

Mrs. ELLMERS. How many States would you say that is?

Ms. WACHINO. I think I can give you some State examples. The actual models used by States vary. States have significant flexibility in using things like health homes, the way——

Mrs. ELLMERS. Um-hum.

Ms. WACHINO [continuing]. Missouri did——

Mrs. ELLMERS. Um-hum.

Ms. WACHINO [continuing]. Where they saw improvements in clinical outcomes and reductions in costs.

Mrs. ELLMERS. OK.

Ms. WACHINO. So I can give you the examples of models that have worked.

Mrs. ELLMERS. OK. Ms. Yocom, would you like to expand on that as well, or comment on the same from your perspective?

Ms. YOCOM. Well, our work has focused primarily on areas where transparency and better data are important.

Mrs. ELLMERS. Um-hum.

Ms. YOCOM. I think some of CMS' challenges are around not having accurate information with which to gauge the success of the program, and to gauge—to fine tune—where improvements need to be made.

Mrs. ELLMERS. Um-hum. So you see an effort for more transparency and more efficiency and accuracy to be moving forward?

Ms. YOCOM. I think we have seen progress, particularly in efforts to control——

Mrs. ELLMERS. Um-hum.

Ms. YOCOM [continuing]. Improper payments. There——

Mrs. ELLMERS. So you have seen progress in that area?

Ms. YOCOM. Right.

Mrs. ELLMERS. OK. Great. Ms. Wachino, CMS authorized Federal Medicaid funding in five States for more than 150 State programs.

Based on their names, many of these programs appear to be fully worthwhile causes. However, it is difficult to see how other funded programs promote Medicaid objectives. Let me ask just a few questions. There are a couple States—and I asked Ms. Iritani, when she was with us a couple of days ago—one of these issues, the licensing fees for Oregon, how does that affect patient care in regard to Medicaid? Do you see that as a worthwhile funding issue? Ms.

WACHINO. Congresswoman, it is really important to us that we ensure that the spending we authorize promotes Medicaid objectives. As I had the opportunity to speak to earlier this morning, we have fully responded to many of GAO's recommendations, in terms of wanting to be very clear and straightforward in our approval documents when we determine that a program supports Medicaid objectives. I can't speak to the particulars of every program, but I do know that my staff has provided to the committee extensive detail on the programs we——

Mrs. ELLMERS. OK. Well, then, what I will just say, the licensing fees in Oregon, the fishermen's partnership in Massachusetts, and the health workforce retaining in New York, if I can get a response on how those actually are effective measures, that would be great, and I would appreciate it in writing. Thank you.

Ms. WACHINO. I would be happy to do——

Mrs. ELLMERS. And I will yield back, and I now recognize Ms. Schakowsky from Illinois for 5 minutes.

Ms. SCHAKOWSKY. [Inaudible.]

Ms. WACHINO. Yes, thank you for the question. As you spoke to, Medicaid is the Nation's leading source of financing for long-term care in the country. We pay for 64 percent of all nursing home residents in the United States, and we work very actively with States to ensure the quality of nursing home care. Because these are, as you know, very frail—some of the Nation's frailest residents and citizens, people who could have limited mobility, and a lot of complex health needs. We are working not just to ensure quality nursing home care, but also ensuring that people, whenever they are able to, are able to be cared for at homes and in their communities, to really remain active participants in their communities.

Ms. SCHAKOWSKY. I wanted to ask about that. One of the most important elements of long-term care has been community-based care, and that does allow many elderly and disabled to remain in their home, or in assisted living facilities, rather than in institutions. In recent years CMS has worked to reduce its reliance on institutional care and transition individuals to community living. In fact, as you have mentioned earlier today, 51 percent of long-term care spending under Medicaid is spent on community-based services, compared to 10 years ago, when community-based services only made up 33 percent of spending.

So why is it important, as you just said earlier, it—that community-based care be available to Medicaid beneficiaries?

Ms. WACHINO. We hear consistently from beneficiaries that they want to remain in their communities, they want to remain active, and they want to remain with their families as much as possible. And we are lucky to have a number of tools in the Medicaid program to help support that. Things like home and community-based waivers, and giving beneficiaries the ability to self-direct their care, to hire their direct service workers, and to fire their direct care service workers if they are not happy. And if you look across the States, we see nearly every State is moving forward with some option.

But the proof is in the pudding, as you say, and seeing the equalization of spending on institutional care versus home, community-based care is a very major advance in modernization in our program, and we are going to keep at it, and move the needle further.

Ms. SCHAKOWSKY. All right. And, finally, as you mentioned in your testimony, since the beginning of ACA's first enrollment period, 12.3 million people have gained coverage through Medicaid or CHIP. According to The Urban Institute, the current uninsured rate nationwide for nonelderly adults is 10 percent down—10 percent, which is down from 17.8 percent, before the implementation of the ACA. Even more impressive, States have expanded Medicaid—that have expanded Medicaid have an uninsured rate of 7.5 percent compared to 14.4 percent in States that have not expanded Medicaid. Can you explain how Medicaid expansion helped to drastically reduce the uninsured rate?

Ms. WACHINO. Well, I think we know that many low-income Americans fall into the coverage gap that is created when States have expanded Medicaid, and one of the things that we can do as a country to make further advances in covering the uninsured, and to see even progress beyond what you have just described is to work with States on Medicaid expansion. And we are very committed to working with every State to finding an approach that provides its lowest-income citizens access to needed health care so we could start improving their quality, and so that those people can benefit.

Ms. SCHAKOWSKY. It seems to me the Medicaid expansion, because it was so public, also helped other enrollment, that people became more aware of Medicaid, so I think it even went beyond the new population.

Ms. WACHINO. That is right. The benefits of expansion go beyond the newly eligible population because States that cover Medicaid expansion are able to convey a clear message to their lowest-income residents that you are eligible for coverage. And we know that when there is that message, eligible people come and enroll, and get the health care they need.

Ms. SCHAKOWSKY. Thank you so much. I yield back.

Mrs. ELLMERS. The gentlelady yields back. And, with that, I think we are finishing up. I would like to thank our panel for being with us today. I would like to remind members that they have 10 business days to submit questions for the record. And I will say to the panel, I know there are some very, very specific questions that members are going to be proposing in written form, and we would very much like to have very specific answers to these questions. You know, as we are addressing Medicaid and Medicare issues, we have to remember that these are taxpayer dollars that we are spending, and so we need very specific answers on those questions, and in a prompt fashion, if you can accommodate us on that.

I would like to also say members should submit their questions by the close of business Wednesday, July 22. And, again, thank you very much for being with us today, and to everyone who was here for the hearing. And I call this subcommittee hearing adjourned.

[Whereupon, at 12:33 p.m., the subcommittee was adjourned.]

[Material submitted for inclusion in the record follows:]

PREPARED STATEMENT OF HON. G.K. BUTTERFIELD

Chairman Pitts, thank you for holding this hearing to commemorate the 50th anniversary of Medicaid and to discuss improving health care for vulnerable populations. More than one out of every four people in the eastern North Carolina district I represent live in poverty—it is one of the poorest Congressional districts in the country. Even more alarming is the fact that more than 40 percent of the chil- dren in North Carolina's First District live in poverty. Medicaid is absolutely critical to my constituents. It is especially important to children, since 75 percent of chil- dren who live in poverty in this country depend on Medicaid. The benefits of Med- icaid cannot be overstated—more than 71 million Americans rely on this program. Democrats on this committee have done our part to strengthen Medicaid for mil- lions of Americans.

Many of us here today helped author the Affordable Care Act, which has helped reduce the number of uninsured Americans by 17 million due in large part to Federal support to expand Medicaid.

But many States—like my home of North Carolina—have declined to expand Med- icaid. According to the North Carolina Justice Center, an additional 500,000 North Carolinians would be eligible for Medicaid if our Governor would expand the pro- gram. My State's Governor has blocked more than $2.7 billion in Federal funds that North Carolinians have paid taxes for and rightly deserve. In fact, the North Caro- lina Justice Center estimates that 43,000 jobs would be created in 5 years if our State would expand Medicaid.

The ACA represents the largest step forward for Medicaid since the program's in- ception. Improved transparency, additional safeguards against fraud and abuse, and delivery system reforms have benefitted constituents and saved money. But our work is far from done. I will continue to fight to expand Medicaid in each and every State.

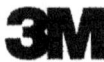

**Energy and Commerce Committee
Subcommittee on Health
Hearing on "Medicaid at 50: Strengthening and Sustaining the Program"
July 8, 2015**

3M Company ("3M") appreciates the opportunity to submit this statement for the record before the Committee on Energy and Commerce, Subcommittee on Health Hearing on "Medicaid at 50: Strengthening and Sustaining the Program."

3M thanks the Committee for its continued efforts to improve all of the critical programs within the health care system to keep pace for the betterment of patients. As the Medicaid program expands and is responsible for more patient lives and health care expenditures, continued oversight of quality, outcomes and cost within the program is essential.

Background on 3M

3M is a large U.S.-based employer and manufacturer established over a century ago in Minnesota. Today, 3M is one of the largest and most diversified manufacturing companies in the world. We are a global company conducting the majority of our manufacturing and research activities in the United States.

3M, formerly known as Minnesota Mining and Manufacturing, is an American company currently headquartered in St Paul, Minnesota. The company, created in 1902 by a small group of entrepreneurs, initially began as a small sandpaper product manufacturer. Today, 3M is one of the largest and most diversified manufacturing companies in the world. 3M is home to such well-known brands as Scotch, Scotch-Brite, Post-it®, Nexcare®, Filtrete®, Command®, and Thinsulate® and is composed of five business sectors: Consumer; Electronics and Energy; Industrial; Health Care; and Safety and Graphics.

Ahead of their peers, 3M's founders insisted on a robust investment in R&D. Looking back, it is this early and consistent commitment to R&D that has been the main component of 3M's success. Today, 3M maintains 46 different technology platforms. These diverse platforms allow 3M scientists to share and combine technologies from one business to another, creating unique, innovative solutions for its customers. The financial commitment to R&D equated to $1.7 billion of R&D spending in 2013 and over $7.6 billion over the last 5 years. These investments produced high quality jobs for 4400 researchers in the United States. The results are equally impressive with 625 U.S. patents awarded in 2014 alone, and over 40,000 global patents and patent applications.

3M's worldwide sales in 2014 were $31 billion. 3M is one of the 30 companies on the Dow Jones Average and is a component of the Standard & Poor's 500 Index. This success is attributable to the people of 3M. Generations of imaginative and industrious employees in all of its business sectors throughout the world have built 3M into a successful global company.

3M: Health Information Systems

3M Health Information Systems works with providers, payers and government agencies to anticipate and navigate a changing healthcare landscape. 3M provides healthcare data aggregation, analysis, and strategic services that help clients move from volume to value-based health care, resulting improved provider performance and better patient outcomes. 3M HIS is one of the industry leaders in computer-assisted coding, clinical documentation improvement, performance monitoring, quality outcomes reporting and terminology management.

Targeting the Problem to Improve Quality and Reduce Costs

The 2012 Institute of Medicine (IOM) study *Best Care at Lower Cost* estimated that unneeded services, mistakes, delivery system ineffectiveness and missed prevention opportunities were leading to $395 billion in annual healthcare expenditures that could be avoided without worsening health outcomes.

If the health care system can focus on targeting these unneeded services, mistakes, inefficiencies and missed opportunities, we can improve patient care and save valuable health care resources.

We know that failures in quality typically result in a need for more interventions to correct the quality problem resulting in high rates of potentially preventable:

- Complications,
- Readmissions,
- Admissions,
- Emergency room visits, and
- Outpatient procedures and diagnostic tests.

These five potentially preventable events, or PPEs, identify an underlying quality of care problem. They also represent a large proportion of the unnecessary spending within our health care system and should be the target of state and federal efforts to make our system more efficient and effective for patients and tax payers. We can improve our health care system if we can reduce PPEs through better quality, efficiency, and care coordination.

State Efforts to Improve Outcomes and Reduce Costs in Their Medicaid Programs

For most states, expenditures for Medicaid are one of the largest or the largest item in the state budget. This has necessitated that states seek innovative ways to control Medicaid expenditures. **These successful payment system reforms are practical, transparent, and identify opportunities for improvement that are being realized today.**

Leading Medicaid programs have focused on payment system reforms that link the outcomes of care to payment. These state programs are boldly leading the way on healthcare system payment reform as they respond to their urgent state budget issues. States like Maryland, New York, and Texas have adopted payment systems that create clear financial incentives for providers to increase efficiency and improve quality outcomes.

The payment reforms implemented by state Medicaid programs have been more comprehensive than those implemented by Medicare. Examples include outcomes focused pay for performance programs that target a wider range of clinically-related readmissions and a more comprehensive set of healthcare acquired complications than is currently included in Medicare payment policies.

Several state Medicaid agencies are in the process of implementing comprehensive outcomes payment reforms. In Texas, Senate Bill 7 was passed in 2011 to establish an outcomes payment adjustment across all healthcare delivery organizations including managed care plans. Similarly, New York issued regulations that establish comprehensive outcomes based payment reform. In its first three years, a potentially preventable complication payment adjustment system in Maryland has resulted in a 32 percent reduction in inpatient complications. In Minnesota, the first three years of a potentially preventable readmissions project has resulted in a 20 percent reduction in readmissions. Key components of these state level reforms were contained in H.R. 5823, the "Incentivizing Health Care Quality Outcomes Act of 2014."

While some of the implementation details across these state Medicaid reforms may differ, they all have the following characteristics in common:

- Payment adjustments for quality are based on the outcomes of care
- Measureable and clinically meaningful objectives for improving the outcomes of care are established
- Comprehensive provider specific information on the outcomes of care are made publically available

The core objective of an outcomes payment reform is to motivate provider behavioral change that leads to improved outcomes, better quality and lower costs. Outcomes related payment adjustments are directed at health delivery organizations with a consistently higher risk-adjusted rates of PPEs because they are more likely to have underlying quality problems that can be identified and corrected. By focusing on outcomes that are potentially preventable, healthcare delivery organizations can direct their quality improvement efforts on problems where quality can actually be improved.

As an inherent byproduct of responding to the financial incentives in an outcomes payment reform, healthcare delivery organizations must find new and innovative ways to coordinate care and improve quality. Because there is a clear and unambiguous relationship between each PPE and its financial consequences, reductions in the rate of PPEs directly translate into lower cost of care. The only way to significantly improve outcomes performance is to provide better care coordination and improved quality. As a result, the care for patients will improve as healthcare delivery organizations strive to improve their outcome performance.

Conclusion: We Should Learn from What is Working

It is imperative that we learn from state Medicaid program efforts that are fully operational and producing real results. A more widespread adoption of these innovative payment system reforms across entire Medicaid program should encouraged. Payment system reforms that are practical, transparent, and identify opportunities for improvement can yield better outcomes at lower costs. We should apply such successful concepts not only across the Medicaid program but also to Medicare as well.

We would appreciate the opportunity to present additional findings and would welcome the opportunity to answer any questions. Please contact Megan Ivory Carr at mmivory@mmm.com or 202.414.3000 for any information.

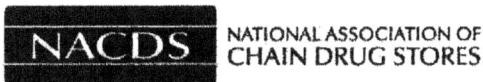

Statement

Of

The National Association of Chain Drug Stores

For

U.S. House of Representatives
Energy and Commerce Committee

Subcommittee on Health

Hearing on

"Medicaid at 50: Strengthening and Sustaining the Program"

July 8, 2015
10:15 a.m.
2322 Rayburn House Office Building

National Association of Chain Drug Stores (NACDS)
1776 Wilson Blvd., Suite 200
Arlington, VA 22209
703-549-3001
www.nacds.org

As Congress examines how to strengthen and sustain the Medicaid program, the National Association of Chain Drugs Stores (NACDS) is writing to offer our support for those efforts and how retail pharmacy can play a role in those efforts. NACDS represents traditional drug stores and supermarkets and mass merchants with pharmacies – from regional chains with four stores to national companies. Chains operate more than 40,000 pharmacies, and employ more than 3.2 million individuals, including 179,000 pharmacists. They fill over 2.9 billion prescriptions yearly, and help patients use medicines correctly and safely, while offering innovative services that improve patient health and healthcare affordability.

Pharmacists play a vital role in advancing the health, safety, and well-being of Medicaid beneficiaries. As the face of neighborhood healthcare, community pharmacies and pharmacists provide access to Medicaid prescription medications and over the counter products, as well as cost-effective health services such as immunizations and disease screenings for Medicaid beneficiaries. Through personal interactions with Medicaid beneficiaries, face-to-face consultations, and convenient access to preventive care services, local pharmacists are helping to shape the future of the Medicaid program – in partnership with doctors, nurses and others. Accordingly, as Congress examines the future of Medicaid, it is critical that Congress acts to prevent potentially harmful alterations to the Medicaid drug benefit. Doing so would ensure that community pharmacies can continue to offer positive and valuable health care services and benefits to Medicaid beneficiaries

The Value of Community Pharmacy to the Medicaid Program

Community pharmacies offer millions of Medicaid beneficiaries across the country innovative programs that deliver unsurpassed value - improving health and wellness and reducing Medicaid costs. Through services such as medication therapy management (MTM), immunization administration, health education, screenings, simple laboratory examinations and procedures, and disease management programs, community pharmacies play an instrumental role in improving overall Medicaid outcomes, patients' quality of life, and the prevention of more costly healthcare treatments for Medicaid beneficiaries.

Community pharmacies offer such value because the pharmacists that they employ are highly educated, trusted healthcare professionals who provide Medicaid patients with important healthcare services. In recent years, community pharmacists have played an increasingly important role in the care of Medicaid beneficiaries, providing convenient, accessible, and cost-effective health services and working in partnership with healthcare entities and other providers to improve health outcomes.

Not only are community pharmacists well-qualified and highly trusted, but they are also well-situated in local communities, and are often the most readily accessible healthcare provider. Research has shown that nearly all Americans (94%) live within five miles of a community retail pharmacy. Such convenient access is vital to reaching Medicaid beneficiaries who often have difficult with transportation for their healthcare needs.

Notably, millions of Medicaid beneficiaries lack adequate and timely access to primary healthcare and this is only expected to worsen as demand increases. Since open enrollment started under the Affordable Care Act (ACA), Medicaid enrollment has grown by 12.3

million. As more and more states adopt the ACA Medicaid expansions, enrollment will exponentially grow placing further strains on the Medicaid healthcare delivery system. Community pharmacies offer an important auxiliary source for Medicaid healthcare services. Notably, the Association of American Medical Colleges projects that by 2020 there will be at least 91,000 fewer doctors than needed to meet demand, and the impact will be most severe on underserved populations, such as Medicaid beneficiaries.

Pharmacists are primed to assist physicians and other healthcare providers with meeting increased demand for Medicaid healthcare services and improving patient outcomes. Highly educated and trained, pharmacists are qualified to perform an expanded set of patient care services, including health testing and chronic care management that are needed by patients - particularly those with chronic conditions. In fact, there is evidence showing that quality of care is improved when pharmacists practice to the fullest extent of their education and training. According to a report issued by the U.S. Public Health Service in 2011, pharmacists involved in the delivery of patient care services, with appropriate privileges across many practice settings, have been successful in improving patient outcomes.

Implementation Timing for AMP-Based FULs

In the near future, the Centers for Medicare and Medicaid Services (CMS) is scheduled to release its Final Rule on Medicaid Covered Outpatient Drugs. By releasing the Final Rule, CMS is expected to finalize the new Medicaid pharmacy reimbursement benchmark known as Average Manufacturer Price (AMP)-based Federal Upper Limits (FULs), as well as the guidance to states for implementing those FULs.

The release of this Final Rule and the timing for states to implement these new AMP-based FULs is a very important issue within the Medicaid program. Implementation of the AMP-based FULs must be done in the proper way to ensure continuing Medicaid beneficiary access to the drugs that they need. Medicaid beneficiary drug access under the AMP-based FULs is tied closely to fair pharmacy reimbursement for a drug's ingredient cost and the cost to dispense. CMS must allow states adequate time to implement AMP-based FULs and adjust corresponding dispensing fees that ensure Medicaid drug reimbursement does not fall below drug acquisition cost and that Medicaid beneficiaries continue to have access to critical prescription drugs.

In particular, the states need adequate time to implement the new AMP-based FULs. Many states face challenging time constraints in quickly introducing legislative and/or regulatory changes to Medicaid drug reimbursement. Many states also face challenging time constraints in performing their own cost of dispensing studies to help determine fair and adequate dispensing fees to correspond with the upcoming changes in ingredient-based drug reimbursement. Moreover, many states will have to file State Plan Amendments with CMS that could also take a number of months to complete and be approved. Accordingly, it is important that CMS provide states with a one year time period to implement the AMP-based FULs once the AMP-based FULs and Final Rule have both been published. As Congress examines the future of Medicaid, we believe that they must keep this timeline in mind regarding their communications with CMS about the future of Medicaid drug reimbursement.

AMPs for Authorized Generics for Purposes of Pharmacy Reimbursement
The House Rules Committee recently introduced proposals to generate funding for the 21st Century Cures Legislation which included a proposal to exclude authorized generic drugs from the calculation of AMPs. The intent of this proposal assumes that removal of authorized generics from the calculation of AMP will increase manufacturer rebates on brand drugs. While this assumption is true, there is a need clarify and ensure that manufacturers continue to meet the requirements and obligations to calculate and report AMPs for authorized generic drugs for rebate and pharmacy reimbursement purposes. Since the Covered Outpatient Drug Rule—which would codify the requirement for manufacturers of authorized generics to report AMPs—is still pending, it is important clarify that AMPs for authorized generics continue to be calculated and reported by manufacturers.

Failure by manufacturers in reporting of authorized generics will result in drastic cuts to pharmacy reimbursement. The lack of reporting of AMPs for authorized generics would mean that one of the higher cost products used to calculate the weighted average for pharmacy reimbursement will be eliminated, resulting in pharmacies being paid below the average acquisition cost of the drug.

On average, the current draft AMP-based FULs, which are based off of AMPs that include authorized generics, already pay pharmacies below cost for over 1/3 of generic drug products. By removing authorized generic drugs from the calculation of AMP and ultimately the calculation of FULs, pharmacy reimbursement will be even lower as a larger number of FULs will fall below pharmacy acquisition costs. These drastic cuts could lead to reduced access to prescription drugs and pharmacy services for Medicaid patients as pharmacies may not be able to withstand these additional financial burdens. As a result, there is the potential for increased overall healthcare expenditures due to the use of more costly healthcare services among Medicaid patients.

We thank you for your leadership on these critically important healthcare issues and look forward to working with you as the nation seeks to address the fiscal challenges before it.

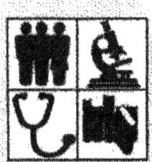

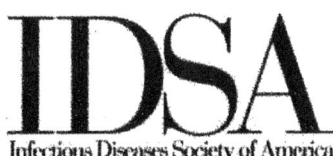

Infectious Diseases Society of America

2014-2015
BOARD OF DIRECTORS

President
Stephen B. Calderwood, MD, FIDSA
Massachusetts General Hospital
Boston, MA

President-Elect
Johan S. Bakken, MD, PhD, FIDSA
St. Luke's ID Associates
Duluth, MN

Vice President
William G. Powderly, MD, FIDSA
Washington University School of Medicine
St. Louis, MO

Secretary
Penelope H. Dennehy, MD, FIDSA
Hasbro Children's Hospital
Providence, RI

Treasurer
Cynthia L. Sears, MD, FIDSA
Johns Hopkins University School of Medicine
Baltimore, MD

Immediate Past President
Barbara E. Murray, MD, FIDSA
The University of Texas Health Science Center
Houston, TX

Judith A. Aberg, MD, FIDSA
Icahn School of Medicine at Mount Sinai
New York, NY

Barbara D. Alexander, MD, MHS, FIDSA
Duke University Medical Center
Durham, NC

R. Michael Buckley, MD, FIDSA
University of Pennsylvania Health System
Philadelphia, PA

Deborah Cotton, MD, MPH, FIDSA
Boston University School of Medicine
Boston, MA

Janet A. Englund, MD, FIDSA
Seattle Children's Hospital
Seattle, WA

Thomas Fekete, MD, FIDSA
Temple University Medical School
Philadelphia, PA

Lawrence P. Martinelli, MD, FIDSA
Covenant Health
Lubbock, TX

Louis B. Rice, MD, FIDSA
Warren Alpert Medical School
of Brown University
Providence, RI

Steven K. Schmitt, MD, FIDSA
Cleveland Clinic
Cleveland, OH

Chief Executive Officer
Mark A. Leasure

IDSA Headquarters
1300 Wilson Boulevard
Suite 300
Arlington, VA 22209
TEL: (703) 299-0200
FAX: (703) 299-0204
EMAIL ADDRESS:
info@idsociety.org
WEBSITE:
www.idsociety.org

July 7, 2015

The Honorable Joe Pitts
Chairman
Subcommittee on Health
Energy and Commerce Committee
U.S. House of Representatives
420 Cannon House Office Building
Washington, DC 20515

The Honorable Gene Green
Ranking Member
Subcommittee on Health
Energy and Commerce Committee
U.S. House of Representatives
2470 Rayburn House Office Building
Washington, DC 20515

Dear Chairman Pitts and Ranking Member Green,

On behalf of the Infectious Diseases Society of America (IDSA), I write to thank you for holding tomorrow's hearing, "Medicaid at 50: Strengthening and Sustaining the Program." The Medicaid program is a critical source of coverage for preventive and health care services for some of our most vulnerable patients. With the Affordable Care Act's (ACA) Medicaid expansion, the program has taken on an even greater role in providing comprehensive and reliable coverage to our patients living with HIV and many others who previously were uninsured. We urge strong and ongoing federal support for this vital program.

I write to offer information and recommendations to strengthen Medicaid reimbursement of infectious diseases (ID) physicians and the impact of ID physician reimbursement on patient care, public health, and research. We hope you will find our perspectives useful as you review this important program and consider improvements.

The Value of the Infectious Diseases (ID) Physician

ID physicians provide expert life-saving care for a wide variety of medically complex patients, including many who rely upon Medicaid for their health coverage. For example, in inpatient hospital settings, ID physicians often consult with the primary treating physician on the care of patients who may have serious infections that require intensive monitoring to accurately diagnose and appropriately manage. ID specialists provide cost-saving stewardship of diagnostic testing. ID specialists optimize treatment by recommending appropriate antibiotics or other antimicrobial drugs, duration of therapy, and route of delivery, and by monitoring clinical and laboratory progress to minimize adverse drug reactions.[1,2] Furthermore, ID specialists facilitate care transitions from the inpatient setting through provision and

---

[1] Petrak RM, et. al. The value of an infectious diseases specialist. *Clin Infect Dis* 2003;36:1013-17.

[2] McQuillen DP, et. al. The value of infectious diseases specialists: non-patient care activities. *Clin Infect Dis* 2008;47:1051-63.

oversight of outpatient antibiotic therapy. Such programs are themselves a form of antimicrobial stewardship; infectious diseases consultation reduced use of parenteral antibiotics by 28% in one study.[3] In outpatient settings, ID physicians routinely provide follow up care to recently hospitalized patients as well as extensive ongoing care to patients with chronic infections such as HIV/AIDS. Of particular note, ID specialists play an important role in the treatment of chronic hepatitis caused by Hepatitis C virus (HCV), which is a disease of high incidence within the Medicaid population and comes with significant treatment costs. Access to ID specialists for patients infected with HCV is critical to ensure that the most appropriate and most cost-effective treatment is provided.

In 2014, several IDSA leaders published, "Infectious Diseases Specialty Intervention Is Associated with Decreased Mortality and Lower Healthcare Costs," in *Clinical Infectious Diseases*.[4] The study reviewed Medicare data from 2008-2009 for over 270,000 hospital stays of patients with at least 1 of 11 targeted serious infections to compare stays that involved ID physician intervention with those that did not, as well as early versus late ID physician intervention. The sample included 101,991 stays with ID physician involvement and 170,366 stays without. Risk adjusted, stays with ID physician involvement were associated with significantly lower rates of mortality and 30-day readmission rates. Patients receiving care from an ID physician also had significantly lower risk-adjusted lengths of hospital stay, far fewer intensive care unit (ICU) days, and much lower Medicare charges and payments than those who did not receive any ID physician care. Patients receiving early intervention from an ID physician (within 2 days of admission) had even better outcomes as compared to those with no ID physician involvement: 3.8% shorter overall hospital stays, 5.1% shorter ICU stays, 3.4% lower costs for the hospital stay, and 6.2% lower costs for the 30 days post-discharge. Although these findings are based solely upon Medicare data, we believe the impact of care from an ID physician is applicable across patient populations and payers, including Medicaid.

ID physicians provide tremendous value beyond direct patient care as well. For example, ID physicians contribute significantly to our national security, leading public health responses to natural and manmade ID threats such as bioterrorism attacks, Middle East Respiratory Syndrome Coronavirus (MERS-CoV), Ebola virus disease, antibiotic resistance, foodborne illnesses, and other emerging threats. ID physicians provide critical expertise and leadership for infection control programs and activities at healthcare facilities across the nation. ID physicians are also leading antibiotic stewardship programs at institutions throughout the country, which are critically needed to optimize patient care and outcomes and curtail the overuse and misuse of antibiotics that is driving the development of resistance. As the federal government pursues the establishment of stewardship programs in all hospitals and long-term care facilities (as indicated in the National Action Plan for Combating Antibiotic Resistant Bacteria), we will rely upon a well-trained cadre of ID physicians to direct this important effort at the local and institutional level. Further, ID physicians are critical for the conduct of clinical trials to evaluate and

---

[3] Shrestha, NK et. al. Antimicrobial stewardship at transition of care from hospital to community. *Infect Control Hosp Epidemiol.* 2012 Apr;33(4):401-4. doi: 10.1086/664758.

[4] Schmitt, Steven et. al. Infectious Diseases Specialty Intervention Is Associated With Decreased Mortality and Lower Healthcare Costs. *Clin Infect Dis.* (2014) 58 (1): 22-28.

validate greatly needed new vaccines, diagnostics, and antibiotics and other antimicrobial drugs. We greatly appreciate this Subcommittee's leadership in advancing the 21st Century Cures Act (H.R. 6), which IDSA is proud to support. And we underscore that the success of provisions in this bill seeking to stimulate urgently needed antibiotic research and development will hinge upon the availability of ID physicians to conduct the necessary clinical trials.

The Future of ID Patient Care, Public Health, and Research in Peril

Unfortunately, despite the vital role of ID physicians in caring for patients, protecting public health and driving research, the future of this specialty is in jeopardy as fewer and fewer young physicians are choosing to enter this field. Data from the National Residency Match Program (NRMP) indicate a disturbing decline in the number of individuals entering into ID fellowship training. In the 2010-2011 academic year, there were 342 NRMP applicants matching nationwide in ID. This number has consistently declined every year since, with only 276 applicants matching via the NRMP in 2014-2015. Interestingly, ID and nephrology are the only two internal medicine subspecialties experiencing this decline. In 2014, IDSA leaders surveyed nearly 600 internal medicine residents about their career choices. While results have not yet been published, we can share that very few residents self-identified as planning to go into ID. A far higher number reported that they were interested in ID, but chose another field instead. Among that group, salary was the most often cited reason for not choosing ID.

Reimbursement for ID Physicians

Relatively low compensation for ID physicians as compared to other medical specialties is an important concern for IDSA, and one that we hope the Subcommittee will examine closely. Over 90% of the care provided by ID physicians is considered evaluation and management (E&M), as opposed to procedures. The face-to-face encounters that ID physicians have with patients suffering from serious infections continue to be undervalued by current payment systems that much more generously reward procedures. To elaborate, infectious diseases specialists often treat patients with complex, severe infections that require strict adherence to antimicrobial treatment protocols that may last several weeks to months. Moreover, it is not uncommon that patients with severe infections have multiple co-morbidities that bring added complexity to their management and treatment. ID specialist-managed patients infected with HIV and HCV require ongoing care coordination. The provision of these E&M services requires a high level of expertise and complex medical decision-making that is inappropriately undervalued under current payment systems, including Medicaid.

The inappropriate undervaluing of E&M services has created a significant compensation disparity between ID physicians and specialists who provide more procedure-based care, as well as primary care physicians who provide similar or identical E&M services but who receive payment increases simply because they are called "primary care physicians." This disparity is a key driver of the waning interest in ID among young physicians. For example, a 2015 review by Medscape of 26 medical specialties found that ID was 6th from the bottom.[5] Average annual

---

[5] Peckham, Carol. Medscape Infectious Disease Physician Compensation Report 2015.

salaries for ID physicians are only 8.7% higher than the average salary of general internal medicine physicians, even though ID certification requires an additional 2-3 years of training. While we recognize that physician compensation is still significantly higher than what most Americans earn, we are nonetheless tremendously concerned about the future of the ID specialty, the patients who will need access to care for serious or life-threatening infections, and public health activities that will continue to rely upon ID physician expertise and leadership. Far too few young physicians are pursuing ID careers, instead seeking the higher compensation associated with other specialties whose annual salaries are 1 2/3 to twice that of ID specialists. The significant debt burden facing young physicians ($200,000 on average for the class of 2014) is understandably driving many individuals toward more profitable specialties.

Recommendations

Medicaid policy is one area in which the federal government can help address the payment disparity facing ID physicians. For example, the ACA currently provides for increased reimbursement for physicians who perform primary care services to Medicare beneficiaries and who are of a specific designation, (e.g., family medicine, internal medicine, geriatric medicine, or pediatric medicine). It is important to understand there is no code in the physician fee schedule for "primary care services." Primary care physicians (PCPs) and infectious diseases specialists bill identical E&M codes, and both coordinate care for individual patients. However, because of how the legislation was drafted, an ID specialist will be reimbursed less than other physicians for providing the same or usually substantially more complex E&M services. IDSA continues to advocate for appropriate reimbursement for these face-to-face patient encounters provided by ID physicians within the Medicare program. As the Subcommittee examines broad issues regarding the Medicaid program, we are hopeful that you can consider opportunities to provide adequate reimbursement for E&M services, including those provided by ID physicians.

The ACA also included a provision that provided Medicare-level reimbursement rates under Medicaid to physicians practicing in the specialties of family medicine, pediatrics, and internal medicine as well as related pediatric and internal medicine subspecialists, including ID physicians. While not a comprehensive solution to ID physician reimbursement concerns, this policy was helpful, particularly in allowing ID physicians to maintain or expand their Medicaid patient populations. We understand that Congress opted to allow this provision to expire at the end of 2014 and that a variety of complex factors led to that decision. However, we urge the Subcommittee to consider ways to address ID physician reimbursement as you consider broader Medicaid policies. We also recognize that Medicaid policy alone cannot thoroughly and sufficiently address concerns regarding ID physician compensation and the decreasing numbers of people entering this important field. We look forward to other opportunities to engage with the subcommittee on these issues and offer additional policy recommendations for your consideration.

PAGE FIVE—IDSA Letter to E&C Health Subcommittee Leadership RE Medicaid Hearing

Once again, we thank the Subcommittee for holding this important hearing, and look forward to continuing to work with you on issues of importance to patients and public health. Should you have any questions, please feel free to contact Amanda Jezek, IDSA's Vice President for Public Policy and Government Relations at ajezek@idsociety.org or 703-740-4790.

Sincerely,

Stephen B. Calderwood, MD, FIDSA
President, IDSA

IDSA represents over 10,000 infectious diseases physicians and scientists devoted to patient care, disease prevention, public health, education, and research in the area of infectious diseases. Our members care for patients of all ages with serious infections, including meningitis, pneumonia, tuberculosis, HIV/AIDS, antibiotic-resistant bacterial infections such as those caused by methicillin-resistant Staphylococcus aureus (MRSA), vancomycin-resistant enterococci (VRE), and Gram-negative bacterial infections such as Acinetobacter baumannii, Klebsiella pneumoniae, and Pseudomonas aeruginosa, emerging infections such as Middle East respiratory syndrome coronavirus (MERS-CoV), Enterovirus D68, and Ebola virus disease, and bacteria containing novel resistance mechanisms such as the New Delhi metallo-beta-lactamase (NDM) enzymes and others that make them resistant to a broad range of antibacterial drugs, including one of our most powerful classes of antibiotics, the carbapenems (carbapenem-resistant Enterobacteriaceae, or CRE).

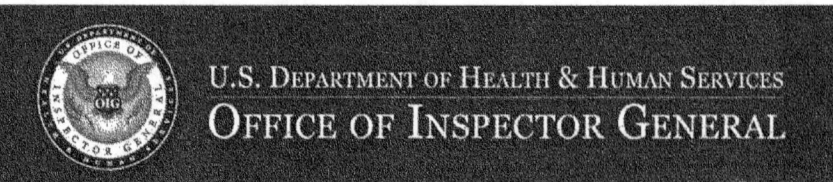

U.S. DEPARTMENT OF HEALTH & HUMAN SERVICES

OFFICE OF INSPECTOR GENERAL

Statement for the Record for the

United States House of Representatives

Committee on Energy and Commerce

Subcommittee on Health

"Medicaid at 50: Recommendations to Improve
the Efficiency and Effectiveness of the Program"

Statement from:

Office of Inspector General
Department of Health and Human Services

July 8, 2015

109

Statement of
Office of Inspector General
Department of Health and Human Services

In 1975, the Medicaid program provided coverage to approximately 20 million beneficiaries at a cost of $12.6 billion.[1] One year later, the Department of Health and Human Services (HHS or the Department) Office of Inspector General (OIG) was established. Now, thirty-nine years later, Medicaid covers approximately 70 million beneficiaries[2] at a cost of $438 billion and makes up a significant portion of OIG's oversight and enforcement work.[3] Over that time, the Medicaid program has expanded from covering the medical expenses for specific categories of individuals, e.g., individuals with disabilities and dependent children receiving public assistance, to a program that now serves as the nation's largest source for public health coverage for a wide range of beneficiaries.

Considering the vital and growing role that Medicaid plays in the nation's health care system, OIG understands how important it is to ensure that both the Centers for Medicare & Medicaid Services (CMS) and the States jointly operate a Medicaid program that is effective and efficient and delivers high-quality health care to its beneficiaries. To that end, OIG continues to make oversight of the Medicaid program a critically important piece of our mission to protect the integrity of HHS programs and the health and welfare of program beneficiaries. We have identified protecting an expanding Medicaid program from fraud, waste, and abuse as one of the Department's top management and performance challenges.[4]

This statement summarizes significant unimplemented recommendations to improve the efficiency and effectiveness of the Medicaid program. HHS OIG believes that implementation of these recommendations will result in cost savings and/or improvements in the Medicaid program's efficiency and effectiveness.

The recommendations come from OIG audits and evaluations, performed pursuant to the Inspector General Act of 1978, as amended. These recommendations were recently released in OIG's March 2015 *Compendium of Unimplemented Recommendations* (Compendium). For more information about these and other unimplemented recommendations please see the full 2015 Compendium available at: http://oig.hhs.gov/reports-and-publications/compendium/index.asp

OIG is committed to working with CMS, the States, Congress, and other stakeholders to ensure that the Medicaid program operates as efficiently and effectively as possible so that Medicaid beneficiaries receive high quality health care services.

---

[1] CMS, *2013 Actuarial Report on the Financial Outlook for Medicaid*, available at https://www.cms.gov/Research-Statistics-Data-and-Systems/Research/ActuarialStudies/downloads/MedicaidReport2010.pdf
[2] CMS, *Medicaid & CHIP, April 2015 Monthly Applications, Eligibility Determinations and Enrollment Report*, available at http://medicaid.gov/medicaid-chip-program-information/program-information/downloads/april-2015-enrollment-report.pdf
[3] Kaiser Family Foundation, *Medicaid & CHIP*, available at http://kff.org/state-category/medicaid-chip/
[4] OIG, *Top Management and Performance Challenges*, available at http://oig.hhs.gov/reports-and-publications/top-challenges/2014/challenge03.asp

OIG Unimplemented Recommendations

High quality, patient-centered care

- ***Ensure that Medicaid children receive all required preventive screening services*** (**Top 25**)[5]
  OIG's review focused on medical, vision, and hearing screenings provided to children under the Early and Periodic Screening, Diagnostic, and Treatment (EPSDT) benefit. We found that very few children received the correct number of vision, hearing, and/or complete medical screenings. Further, we found that children's participation in EPSDT medical screenings remained lower than established goals.

  - CMS should require States to report on vision and hearing screening data for eligible children.

  - CMS should collaborate with States and providers to develop effective strategies to encourage beneficiary participation in screenings.

  CMS concurred with the recommendation and had made efforts to explore adding a requirement and creating a vision quality measure. We continue to monitor CMS's progress in implementing our recommendations. Expected impact is improved quality and safety. OEI-05-08-00520 http://oig.hhs.gov/oei/reports/oei-05-08-00520.pdf

Home and community-based care

- ***Improve oversight of management of Medicaid personal care services*** (**Top 25**)
  OIG's body of work examining personal care services (PCS) has found significant and persistent compliance, payment, and fraud vulnerabilities that demonstrate the need for CMS to take a more active role with States to address these issues. As more and more State Medicaid programs explore home care options like PCS, it is critical that adequate safeguards exist to prevent fraud, waste, and abuse in PCS and other important home care benefits.

  OIG made several recommendations to improve CMS's oversight of PCS:

  - Promulgate regulations to reduce significant variation in States' personal care services laws and regulations by creating or expanding Federal requirements and issuing operational guidance for claims documentation, beneficiary assessments, plans of care, and supervision of attendants.

---

[5] Top 25 indicates that the unimplemented recommendation is included in OIG's Top 25 unimplemented recommendations that, on the basis of the professional opinion of OIG, would best protect the integrity of HHS programs if implemented. OIG is required by law to report the Top 25 unimplemented recommendations in the Compendium. For more information on the Top 25 unimplemented recommendations, see our 2015 Compendium at http://oig.hhs.gov/reports-and-publications/compendium/files/compendium2015.pdf

111

- Promulgate regulations to reduce significant variation in State PCS attendant qualification standards and the potential for beneficiary exposure to unqualified PCS attendants by establishing minimum Federal qualification standards applicable to all PCS reimbursed by Medicaid.

- Promulgate regulations to improve CMS's and States' ability to monitor billing and care quality by requiring States to (1) either enroll all PCS attendants as providers or require all PCS attendants to register with the State Medicaid agencies and assign each attendant a unique identifier and (2) require that PCS claims include the specific date(s) when services were performed and the identities of the rendering PCS attendants.

- Issue guidance to States regarding adequate prepayment controls. Consider whether additional controls are needed to ensure that PCS are allowed under program rules and are provided.

- Take action to provide States with data suitable for identifying overpayments for PCS claims during periods when beneficiaries are receiving institutional care paid for by Medicare or Medicaid.

CMS concurred with the recommendation. In June 2014, CMS indicated that it promulgated final rules for the new Community First Choice benefit, under section 1915(k) and for home- and community-based services (HCBS) provided under sections 1915(c) and 1915(i) of the Social Security Act. OIG believes CMS's actions do not fully implement the recommendation. We recommended that CMS promulgate regulations to reduce variation in State rules regarding PCS by creating Federal requirements for claims documentation, beneficiary assessments, plans of care, and supervision of attendants. The final rules address beneficiary assessments and plan-of-care provisions. However, they do not address provisions related to consistent claims documentation and supervision of attendants. We continue to monitor CMS's progress in implementing our recommendations. Expected impact is an estimated savings of $1.3 billion and improved program management. OIG-12-12-01 http://oig.hhs.gov/reports-and-publications/portfolio/portfolio-12-12-01.pdf

Other OIG significant unimplemented recommendations:
- Require at least one onsite visit before a home and community-based services waiver program is renewed and develop detailed protocols for such visit. CMS concurred with this recommendation in part. OEI-02-08-00170 http://oig.hhs.gov/oei/reports/oei-02-08-00170.pdf

- Make information available to the public about State compliance with the home and community-based services waiver assurances available to the public. CMS concurred with this recommendation. OEI-02-08-00170 http://oig.hhs.gov/oei/reports/oei-02-08-00170.pdf

Medicaid managed care

- *Strengthen Oversight of State access standards for Medicaid Managed Care* (Top 25)

  OIG reviewed State standards and oversight related to Medicaid managed care organizations' (MCO) maintenance of a sufficient network of providers to provide adequate access to care for enrollees. We found that State standards for access to care vary widely and that CMS provides limited oversight of these standards. Additionally, standards are often not specific to certain types of providers or to areas of the State.

  - CMS should strengthen its oversight of State standards and ensure that States develop standards for key providers.

  - CMS should strengthen its oversight of State's methods to assess plan compliance and ensure that States conduct direct tests of access standards.

  - CMS should improve States' efforts to identify and address violations of access standards and provide technical assistance and share effective practices.

  CMS concurred with the recommendation. In a recent notice of proposed rulemaking,[6] CMS proposed new regulatory requirements to improve and monitor beneficiary access to care in the Medicaid MCO setting. We continue to monitor CMS's progress in implementing our recommendations. Expected impact is improved quality and safety. OEI-02-11-00320 http://oig.hhs.gov/oei/reports/oei-02-11-00320.pdf

  Other OIG significant unimplemented recommendations:
- Work with States to assess the number of providers offering appointments and improve the accuracy of plan information. CMS concurred with this recommendation. OEI-02-13-00670 http://oig.hhs.gov/oei/reports/oei-02-13-00670.pdf

- Work with States to ensure that plans' networks are adequate and meet the needs of their Medicaid managed care enrollees. CMS concurred with this recommendation. OEI-02-13-00670 http://oig.hhs.gov/oei/reports/oei-02-13-00670.pdf

- Require that State contracts with managed care entities include methods to verify with beneficiaries whether services billed by providers were received. CMS concurred with this recommendation. OEI-01-09-00550 http://oig.hhs.gov/oei/reports/oei-01-09-00550.pdf

Data systems

- *Improve the Transformed Medicaid Statistical Information System* (Top 25)

---

[6] 80 Fed. Reg. 31098 (Jun. 1, 2015), available at http://www.gpo.gov/fdsys/pkg/FR-2015-06-01/pdf/2015-12965.pdf

113

OIG reviewed CMS's implementation of the Transformed Medicaid Statistical Information System (T-MSIS) that is designed to operate as a national database of Medicaid and Children's Health Insurance Program (CHIP) information to cover a broad range of user needs, including program integrity. We found that some progress had been made in 12 volunteer States; however, most other States had not started implementing T-MSIS, and they reported varied timeframes for when they planned to begin. Furthermore, early T-MSIS implementation outcomes raised questions about the completeness and accuracy of T-MSIS data upon national implementation.

- CMS should ensure that the national T-MSIS is complete, accurate, and timely.

- CMS should ensure that States submit required T-MSIS data and establish a deadline for when national T-MSIS data will be available.

CMS concurred with the recommendation. In March 2014, CMS indicated that it is working to create a set of rules to govern the submission of T-MSIS data. CMS also indicated that it reviewed States' source-to-target mapping documents and distributed State technical requirements. In addition, CMS plans to define State file processing procedures, delineate a data quality oversight strategy, and provide stakeholders with information on data quality issues. OIG has ongoing work[7] that will assess the completeness of States' submission of T-MSIS data. We continue to monitor CMS's progress in implementing our recommendations. Expected impact is improved program management. OEI-05-12-00610 http://oig.hhs.gov/oei/reports/oei-05-12-00610.pdf

Other OIG significant unimplemented recommendations:
- Require each State Medicaid agency to report all terminated providers. CMS concurred with this recommendation. OEI-06-12-00031 http://oig.hhs.gov/oei/reports/oei-06-12-00031.pdf

- Ensure that the shared information contains only records that meet CMS's criteria for inclusion. CMS concurred with this recommendation. OEI-06-12-00031 http://oig.hhs.gov/oei/reports/oei-06-12-00031.pdf

- Work with States to improve the quality of claims data for drugs submitted by providers and pharmacies. CMS concurred with this recommendation. OEI-05-11-00580 http://oig.hhs.gov/oei/reports/oei-05-11-00580.pdf

- Help States obtain better data on ineligible drugs. CMS concurred with this recommendation. OEI-05-11-00580 http://oig.hhs.gov/oei/reports/oei-05-11-00580.pdf

- Facilitate States' submission of standardized claims data. CMS concurred with this recommendation. OEI-05-11-00580 http://oig.hhs.gov/oei/reports/oei-05-11-00580.pdf

[7] OEI-05-15-00050; expected issue date: fiscal year 2016

- CMS should be more engaged in dispute resolution between States and drug manufactures. CMS concurred in part with this recommendation. OEI-05-11-00580 http://oig.hhs.gov/oei/reports/oei-05-11-00580.pdf

Program integrity and financial management

- ***Ensure that States calculate accurate costs for Medicaid services provided by local public providers.* (Top 25)**
  OIG's review focused State practices that utilize the Federal Upper Payment Limit (UPL) to obtain Federal Medicaid funds without committing the States' shares of required matching funds or by other means artificially inflate the Federal share. We found that some States utilized the UPL rules to their advantage by requiring certain classes of facilities to transfer the UPL funds to the States to be put to other uses, leaving the facilities underfunded.

  - CMS should provide States with definitive guidance for calculating the UPL, which should include using facility-specific UPLs that are based on actual cost report data.

  - CMS should require that the return of Medicaid payments by a county or local government to the State be declared a refund of those payments and thus be used to offset the Federal share generated by the original payment.

  In 2008, CMS issued a final rule that, among other things, would limit Medicaid payments to public providers to their costs of providing care, but the rule was ultimately vacated by Federal District Court. We continue to monitor CMS's progress in implementing our recommendations. Expected impact is estimated savings of $3.87 billion over 5 years and improved payment efficiency. A-03-00-00216 http://oig.hhs.gov/oas/reports/region3/30000216.pdf

  Other OIG significant unimplemented recommendations:
- Ensure that all States appropriately report offset drug rebate amounts. CMS concurred with this recommendation. OEI-03-12-00520 https://oig.hhs.gov/oei/reports/oei-03-12-00520.pdf

- Seek legislative authority to extend the additional rebate provisions for brand-name drugs to generic drugs. CMS agreed to consider this recommendation. A-06-07-00042 http://oig.hhs.gov/oas/reports/region6/60700042.pdf

- Work with State Medicaid agencies to determine whether the use of manufacturer rebates and lower provider reimbursement rates could achieve net savings for the purchase of diabetes test strips. CMS concurred with this recommendation. A-05-13-00033 http://oig.hhs.gov/oas/reports/region5/51300033.pdf

- Encourage States to adopt a multitiered payment system to bring pharmacy reimbursement more in line with the actual acquisition cost of drug products. CMS

concurred in part with this recommendation. A-06-02-
00041 http://oig.hhs.gov/oas/reports/region6/60200041.pdf

- Take action to provide States with data suitable for identifying overpayments for PCS claims during periods when beneficiaries are receiving institutional care paid for by Medicare or Medicaid. OIG 12-12-01. CMS concurred with this recommendation. http://oig.hhs.gov/reports-and-publications/portfolio/portfolio-12-12-01.pdf

116

HealthAffairs

At the Intersection of Health, Health Care and Policy

Cite this article as:
Sayeh Nikpay, Thomas Buchmueller and Helen Levy
Early Medicaid Expansion In Connecticut Stemmed The Growth In Hospital
Uncompensated Care
Health Affairs, 34, no.7 (2015):1170-1179

doi: 10.1377/hlthaff.2015.0107

The online version of this article, along with updated information and services, is
available at:
http://content.healthaffairs.org/content/34/7/1170.full.html

For Reprints, Links & Permissions:
    http://healthaffairs.org/1340_reprints.php
E-mail Alerts : http://content.healthaffairs.org/subscriptions/etoc.dtl
To Subscribe: http://content.healthaffairs.org/subscriptions/online.shtml

Health Affairs is published monthly by Project HOPE at 7500 Old Georgetown Road, Suite 600,
Bethesda, MD 20814-6133. Copyright © 2015 by Project HOPE - The People-to-People Health
Foundation. As provided by United States copyright law (Title 17, U.S. Code), no part of *Health
Affairs* may be reproduced, displayed, or transmitted in any form or by any means, electronic or
mechanical, including photocopying or by information storage or retrieval systems, without prior
written permission from the Publisher. All rights reserved.

Not for commercial use or unauthorized distribution

Downloaded from content.healthaffairs.org by *Health Affairs* on September 23, 2015
by guest

117

By Sayeh Nikpay, Thomas Buchmueller, and Helen Levy

DOI: 10.1377/hlthaff.2015.0107
HEALTH AFFAIRS 34,
NO. 7 (2015): 1170–1179
©2015 Project HOPE—
The People-to-People Health
Foundation, Inc.

Early Medicaid Expansion In Connecticut Stemmed The Growth In Hospital Uncompensated Care

Sayeh Nikpay (snikpay@umich edu) is a postdoctoral fellow at the Institute for Healthcare Policy and Innovation at the University of Michigan in Ann Arbor and a visiting scholar in the Robert Wood Johnson Foundation Health Policy Scholars Program at the University of California, Berkeley.

Thomas Buchmueller is the Waldo O. Hildebrand Professor of Risk Management and Insurance in the Ross School of Business at the University of Michigan.

Helen Levy is a research associate professor at the Institute for Social Research at the University of Michigan.

ABSTRACT As states continue to debate whether or not to expand Medicaid under the Affordable Care Act (ACA), a key consideration is the impact of expansion on the financial position of hospitals, including their burden of uncompensated care. Conclusive evidence from coverage expansions that occurred in 2014 is several years away. In the meantime, we analyzed the experience of hospitals in Connecticut, which expanded Medicaid coverage to a large number of childless adults in April 2010 under the ACA. Using hospital-level panel data from Medicare cost reports, we performed difference-in-differences analyses to compare the change in Medicaid volume and uncompensated care in the period 2007–13 in Connecticut to changes in other Northeastern states. We found that early Medicaid expansion in Connecticut was associated with an increase in Medicaid discharges of 7–9 percentage points, relative to a baseline rate of 11 percent, and an increase of 7–8 percentage points in Medicaid revenue as a share of total revenue, relative to a baseline share of 10 percent. Also, in contrast to the national and regional trends of increasing uncompensated care during this period, hospitals in Connecticut experienced no increase in uncompensated care. We conclude that uncompensated care in Connecticut was roughly one-third lower than what it would have been without early Medicaid expansion. The results suggest that ACA Medicaid expansions could reduce hospitals' uncompensated care burden.

I n debates about the Medicaid expansion in the Affordable Care Act (ACA), hospitals have argued forcefully that expansion would improve their financial position.[1] This argument was not enough to carry the day in all states: As of April 29, 2015, twenty-nine states and the District of Columbia had expanded their Medicaid programs.[2] In several of the remaining states, however, the debate about whether (or how) to expand Medicaid continues.

Multiple analysts have projected that one consequence of Medicaid expansion will be a reduction in the uncompensated care costs faced by hospitals.[3-5] Some early evidence suggests that Medicaid expansion has indeed reduced uncompensated hospital care. A recent report from the Department of Health and Human Services explored aspects of Medicaid expansion using data from five large for-profit hospital chains operating in both expansion and nonexpansion states and from hospital association surveys in three expansion states.[6] The analysis found that uninsured admissions fell and Medicaid admissions increased, with the largest changes occurring in states that expanded Medicaid under the ACA.

Several other studies also found that coverage

Downloaded from content.healthaffairs.org by Health Affairs on September 23, 2015
by guest

118

expansions and contractions prior to the ACA led to decreases and increases, respectively, in uncompensated care. A recent study showed that significant Medicaid cuts in Tennessee and Missouri in 2005 led to increases in uncompensated care in those states.[7] Another study found that health reform in Massachusetts reduced bad debt (one component of uncompensated care) by 26 percent—a change that reflects the effects of both the state's Medicaid expansion and its implementation of a health insurance exchange.[8]

To estimate the effect of Medicaid expansion—as opposed to Medicaid cuts or to the full package of coverage expansions included in the ACA—on all hospitals, rather than just for-profits, we looked at the experience of Connecticut, a state that expanded its Medicaid program immediately after passage of the ACA.

Prior to the ACA, parents and caretakers with incomes up to 185 percent of the federal poverty level were eligible for Medicaid in Connecticut.[9] Childless adults were eligible for limited medical assistance through the State Administered General Assistance program, a state-financed program with a limited benefit package, if they had incomes below 56 percent of poverty and had less than $1,000 in assets.[10] Higher-income adults who did not have access to affordable group insurance and who experienced difficulty paying nongroup premiums were also able to purchase subsidized coverage through the state-sponsored Charter Oak Health Plan. However, enrollment in this program was declining during our study period because of rising premiums.[11]

As of April 2010, Connecticut offered full Medicaid benefits to childless adults with incomes below 56 percent of poverty, regardless of assets. In contrast with the limited benefits that had been available previously, the full benefits included an expanded provider network as well as long-term care or skilled nursing facility services and home health care benefits.[10] This resulted in 46,000 new Medicaid enrollees by 2014.[12]

Benjamin Sommers and coauthors have shown that Connecticut's decision to expand eligibility in this way led to an increase in Medicaid coverage and a reduction in the number of uninsured among the state's residents.[12] We investigated whether these changes in insurance coverage at the population level translated into an increase in the number of inpatients with Medicaid coverage and a reduction in the amount of uncompensated care provided by hospitals.

Four other states—New Jersey, Washington, Minnesota, and California—and the District of Columbia also chose to expand their Medicaid programs between 2010 and 2014. For various reasons, their experiences do not provide clean natural experiments for investigating the effect of Medicaid expansion on hospital uncompensated care.

New Jersey and Washington used the early opportunity for expansion under the ACA to fund existing state programs without expanding eligibility to new groups. As a result, no increase in insurance coverage was expected.[9] In general, expansions in Medicaid coverage will reduce uncompensated care only to the extent that they reduce the uninsurance rate among hospitalized patients. To the extent that such expansions simply shift patients from one source of public coverage to another, uncompensated care will not change.

Similarly, early expansion did not appear to substantially affect the number of uninsured residents in the District of Columbia. Sommers and coauthors found an insignificant decrease in the uninsurance rate among childless adults, but a significant increase in the uninsurance rate among parents.[12]

Early expansion by California and Minnesota increased the number of people eligible for public insurance and therefore should have had a larger effect on coverage, compared to the situation in states that did not expand eligibility to new groups. However, because California and Minnesota did not implement the expansion until 2011 and because data on hospital uncompensated care are available only with a lag, at this point we have very little post-expansion data on these states.

States that are still deciding whether or not to expand Medicaid need information now on the potential costs and benefits of expansion. Our focus on a single state, Connecticut, offers insights into how expanding Medicaid to cover the uninsured affects hospitals' uncompensated care.

Study Data And Methods

DATA The data we analyzed came from Medicare cost reports for fiscal years 2007–13. These reports are submitted annually by all Medicare-certified hospitals (essentially, all hospitals excluding Veterans Affairs and selected children's hospitals). We combined these annual reports to create a hospital-level data set with up to seven years of data per hospital. The full sample consisted of 30 hospitals in Connecticut and 404 hospitals in the comparison states, providing a total of 1,958 hospital-year observations.

The cost reports include information on the total number of hospital discharges and the number of discharges for certain payer types: Medicaid (Title 19 of the Social Security Act),

Medicare (Title 18), and the Maternal and Child Health program (Title 5). We expected that after 2010 the Medicaid share of discharges would increase in Connecticut, compared to the other states, driven by the increase in childless adults enrolled in Connecticut's Medicaid program. This increase should coincide with a decrease in uninsured discharges. However, to the extent that the early Medicaid expansion caused some people to move from private to public coverage—a phenomenon known as "crowd-out"—private discharges could fall as well.

Unfortunately, the hospital cost reports do not provide separate measures of uninsured and privately insured discharges. Therefore, we could not directly estimate the extent to which the expansion of Medicaid reduced the number of uninsured patients instead of simply crowding out existing private coverage.

One measurable consequence of any decline in the number of uninsured patients should be a decline in uncompensated care. *Uncompensated care* is defined as the sum of charity care and bad debt. Charity care is care for which there was no expectation of payment at the time of discharge, whereas bad debt arises from services for which the hospital billed but did not receive payment. As a practical matter, it is difficult to distinguish these two components of uncompensated care even when they are reported separately, because hospitals vary in their definitions of *charity care*.

It is sometimes argued that the difference between Medicaid reimbursements and the cost of providing care represents a form of uncompensated care. However, such shortfalls are not included in standard definitions of *uncompensated care*[13] or in the measure of uncompensated care reported in the Medicare cost reports.

METHODS It is important to note that starting in 2010, hospitals were required to report data on uncompensated care using more disaggregated categories than had been required previously. For example, hospitals now have to report charity care and bad debt separately and to report charity care amounts by the insurance status of the patient.

. To create a consistent measure of uncompensated care over the study period, and to address the ongoing problem of distinguishing between bad debt and charity care, we aggregated the detailed categories in the post-2010 data to match the pre-2010 measures of uncompensated care. For details on the construction of uncompensated care measures and a comparison with American Hospital Association data, see online Appendix Exhibits 1 and 2.[14]

In the cost reports, uncompensated care is measured in terms of hospital charges. We applied hospital-specific cost-to-charge ratios from

States that are still deciding whether or not to expand Medicaid need information now on the potential costs and benefits of expansion.

the cost reports to construct a measure of the cost of uncompensated care.

We used a difference-in-differences approach to assess the impact of Connecticut's early expansion. Specifically, we investigated whether the change in uncompensated care (or other outcomes of interest, such as the Medicaid share of discharges) after 2010 was larger in Connecticut than in other Northeastern states—specifically, Maine, New Hampshire, New York, Pennsylvania, Rhode Island, and Vermont. The comparison group excluded New Jersey, which as mentioned above was also an ACA early adopter but expanded Medicaid only to people who were previously covered by state and local programs, and Massachusetts, which implemented a major health insurance reform in 2007.

LIMITATIONS Our study and its data had several limitations. One potential limitation of our data is that hospitals often file incomplete information in Medicare cost reports.[15] Although our data contained observations from 94 percent of the hospitals in Connecticut and 86 percent of those in the comparison states, hospital cost reports were sometimes missing information on Medicaid revenues and uncompensated care. To ensure that our results were not biased by sample selection, we tested whether the rate of item nonresponse changed differentially in Connecticut compared to the other states. Although nonresponse was slightly more common in Connecticut overall, the response rate did not change more in Connecticut than in other states after 2010. Thus, there is no reason to expect our estimates to be biased by nonresponse.

As an additional robustness check, we conducted analyses on a subsample of hospitals that were observed continuously over the study period. As we describe below, the results from this balanced panel were very similar to those from the full sample.

Another potential limitation of our analysis is one of external validity: Connecticut's expansion might not be representative of the expansions that are currently under way in other states. One possible reason is that Connecticut used early expansion as an opportunity to expand an existing program, so some enrollees were already insured. However, Connecticut is not alone in this respect. At least fourteen of the states that chose to expand Medicaid in 2014 had some type of program already in place.[12]

Another way in which Connecticut's early experience differs from those of later expansions is that in 2010 Connecticut expanded eligibility to childless adults with incomes only up to 56 percent of poverty, instead of using the 133 percent threshold required by the ACA after 2014. Given the limited nature of the 2010 expansion, we expect the effects of the 2014 expansion to be greater than what we found for Connecticut.

A final limitation of our analysis is that observed reductions in uncompensated care may overstate the improvement in hospitals' financial positions because of the way uncompensated care is measured. Hospitals that treat uninsured patients can count any difference between what those patients pay and the cost of the service as uncompensated care. In contrast, hospitals that treat Medicaid patients cannot count the difference between what Medicaid pays and the cost of the service—the shortfall—as uncompensated care. Therefore, Medicaid expansion would have improved Connecticut hospitals' financial positions only if the state's Medicaid reimbursement rate was higher than what the hospitals would have collected from uninsured people if they had not gained Medicaid eligibility.

The connection between uncompensated care and hospitals' financial position is further complicated by the fact that Connecticut's Medicaid expansion led to some crowding out of existing private coverage.[12] Because private insurers typically reimburse hospitals more generously than state Medicaid programs do, shifts from private coverage to Medicaid would negatively affect Connecticut hospitals' financial positions.

Study Results

Nationally, roughly 58 percent of private hospitals are nonprofit.[16] However, there is much variation across regions, with for-profit hospitals located disproportionately in Southern states.[17] The vast majority of hospitals in our sample were nonprofit: 99 percent of discharges in Connecticut (where only one of thirty hospitals was for-profit) and 90 percent of discharges in the comparison states were from not-for-profit hospitals (Exhibit 1). The sole for-profit hospital in Connecticut did not report information on uncompensated care before expansion.

Average hospital size (measured by numbers of hospital beds) did not differ substantially between facilities in Connecticut and those in the comparison states (Exhibit 1). In terms of baseline market characteristics, the average county-level unemployment rate was similar in Connecticut and the comparison states (6.1 percent versus 6.3 percent).

A comparison of baseline values for our dependent variables also suggests that the other Northeastern states represented a good control group for Connecticut. In 2007–09, Medicaid patients represented 11 percent of discharges in Connecticut and 10 percent in the comparison states (Exhibit 1), although Medicaid represented a smaller share of hospital revenues in Connecticut than in the other states. Uncompensated care as a share of total expenses was 3 percent in both Connecticut and the comparison group.

Exhibit 2 shows trends in Medicaid discharges as a share of total discharges from 2007 through 2013. We used Medicaid discharges during the pre-expansion period (2007–09) as the denominator for calculating this share in both the pre- and post-expansion periods because total discharges could have been affected by Connecticut's expansion.

Sommers and coauthors found a large increase in Medicaid coverage at the population level in Connecticut, relative to neighboring states.[12] This pattern is evident in the hospitalized Connecticut population as well: Medicaid accounted for about the same fraction of discharges in Connecticut and other Northeastern states before 2010, as noted above, but the Medicaid share of discharges nearly doubled in Connecticut after 2010, while it remained approximately unchanged in the other states (Exhibit 2). In 2013, 21 percent of discharges in Connecticut were Medicaid enrollees, compared to 9 percent in the other Northeastern states ($p < 0.01$). Trends in Medicaid revenues show a similar pattern, increasing in Connecticut both in absolute terms and relative to the comparison states (see Appendix Exhibit 3).[14]

There are two channels through which Connecticut's early expansion could have increased the number of Medicaid inpatients: by increasing inpatient utilization among newly insured people and by shifting the source of payment for people who would have been admitted anyway. The second channel includes both patients who otherwise would have been covered by private insurance and those who would have been uninsured. We examined two additional out-

EXHIBIT 1

Descriptive Statistics: Outcome Variables And Characteristics Of Hospitals In 2007–09, Before Medicaid Was Expanded In Connecticut

	Connecticut hospitals		Northeastern hospitals	
	Mean	SD	Mean	SD
OUTCOME VARIABLES, PER HOSPITAL YEAR				
Medicaid discharges				
As share of all discharges	0.11	0.07	0.10	0.08
In levels (weighted)	3,198	3,321	2,463	2,642
Medicaid revenues				
As share of total revenues	0.10	0.03	0.17	0.12
In levels (millions of dollars; weighted average)	135.8	88.1	307.9	441.2
Uncompensated care				
As share of total expenses	0.03	0.02	0.03	0.04
In levels (millions of dollars; weighted average)	13.9	8.8	14.2	18.5
HOSPITAL AND MARKET CHARACTERISTICS				
Organizational status (weighted by discharges)				
Nonprofit	0.99	0.11	0.90	0.30
For profit	0.00	—ᵃ	0.03	0.18
Public	0.01	0.11	0.07	0.25
Total hospital beds	412	209	442	346
County unemployment rate (%)	6.1	1.7	6.3	1.9

SOURCE Authors' analysis of 2007–09 Medicare cost report data. **NOTES** "Northeastern hospitals" are all hospitals in Maine, New Hampshire, New York, Pennsylvania, Rhode Island, and Vermont (the Northeast census region excluding Connecticut and, as explained in the text, New Jersey and Massachusetts). "Uncompensated care" is the sum of charity care and bad debt charges deflated by the cost-to-charge ratio, minus payments from self-pay patients. Results in levels represent the annual average per hospital number of Medicaid discharges, the annual average per hospital amount of Medicaid revenue in millions of dollars; and the annual average per hospital amount of uncompensated care in millions of dollars. All statistics in the table—both shares and levels—are the mean for a hospital year, weighted by average hospital-level discharges in the pre-expansion period. The pre-expansion sample consisted of 646 hospital-year observations from 19 hospitals in Connecticut and 271 hospitals in the Northeast census region for which information on uncompensated care was reported. SD is standard deviation. ᵃThe sole for-profit hospital in Connecticut did not report information on uncompensated care in the pre-expansion period.

EXHIBIT 2

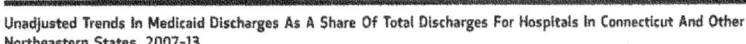

Unadjusted Trends In Medicaid Discharges As A Share Of Total Discharges For Hospitals In Connecticut And Other Northeastern States, 2007–13

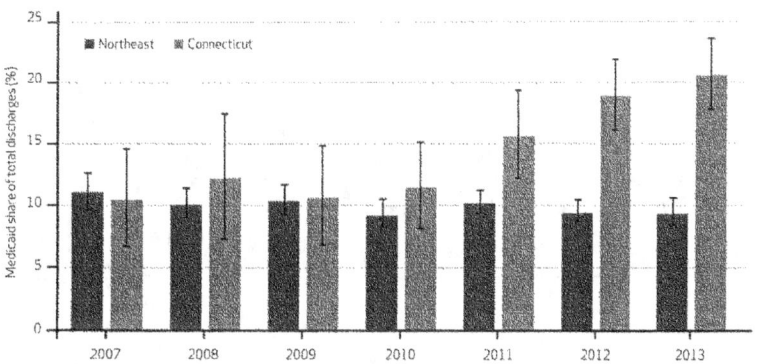

SOURCE Authors' analysis of 2007–13 Medicare cost report data. **NOTES** The analysis sample included 1,985 observations from 434 hospitals in Connecticut and the comparison "Northeastern states" (Maine, New Hampshire, New York, Pennsylvania, Rhode Island, and Vermont). In all years, Medicaid discharges are expressed as a fraction of total discharges in the period before Connecticut expanded Medicaid (2007–09). Error bars represent 95% confidence intervals.

comes to shed light on the relative importance of these two channels. For the results of these examinations, which are summarized below, see Appendix Exhibit 4.[14]

First, we examined trends in total discharges. The results indicated no significant change in Connecticut relative to either the baseline or the change in the other states. This null result for total discharges was consistent with findings from previous studies indicating that the use of inpatient care is relatively insensitive to insurance coverage. The most relevant evidence for our study is from the Oregon Health Insurance Experiment, which found no significant effect of Medicaid coverage on inpatient admissions.[18]

Second, we examined trends in discharges for patients with coverage other than Medicaid, Medicare, or other federal programs. Ideally, we would have looked separately at privately insured and uninsured patients. Unfortunately, as noted above, the Medicare cost reports do not break out these categories. The best we could do was to analyze an "all other" category of discharges for patients not covered by Medicaid or one of the federal programs enumerated in the Medicare cost reports, which included both privately insured and uninsured patients as well as those covered by other state programs.

Looking at this "all other" category, we saw a significant decrease in Connecticut after 2010, relative to the change in other states. In 2013 the fraction of privately insured and uninsured

discharges was 14 percentage points lower in Connecticut than in the comparison states ($p < 0.01$)—a reduction of roughly the same magnitude as the increase in the share of Medicaid discharges. This result further suggests that the main effect of the expansion on hospitals was to change their payer mix instead of increasing their total volume.

Our main interest was in determining whether expanding Medicaid coverage reduced the amount of uncompensated care provided by hospitals. Consistent with national statistics reported by the American Hospital Association,[13] uncompensated care expenditures increased in the comparison nonexpansion states beginning in 2011 (Exhibit 3). In contrast, we saw little change over time in uncompensated care as a fraction of total hospital expenditures in Connecticut. In 2013 uncompensated care as a share of total hospital expenditures was 1.8 percentage points lower in Connecticut than in the comparison states ($p = 0.09$), as a result of the increase in uncompensated care in those states. If we assume that the comparison states represent an appropriate counterfactual, this divergence suggests that Connecticut's decision to expand Medicaid in 2010 fully offset an increase in uncompensated care that the state's hospitals would have faced otherwise.

One question that cannot be answered by our analysis is why uncompensated care in the other Northeastern states increased during this peri-

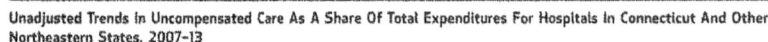

EXHIBIT 3

Unadjusted Trends In Uncompensated Care As A Share Of Total Expenditures For Hospitals In Connecticut And Other Northeastern States, 2007–13

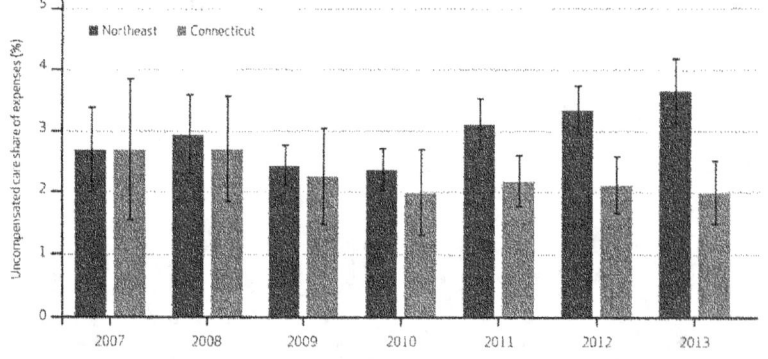

SOURCE Authors' analysis of 2007–13 Medicare cost report data. **NOTES** The analysis sample included 1,985 observations from 434 hospitals in Connecticut and the comparison "Northeastern states" (Maine, New Hampshire, New York, Pennsylvania, Rhode Island, and Vermont). In all years, uncompensated care is expressed as a fraction of total hospital expenditures in the period before Connecticut expanded Medicaid (2007–09). Error bars represent 95% confidence intervals.

od. Anecdotal reports suggest two possibilities. One is the increasing popularity of high-deductible plans,[19,20] and the other is the very slow economic recovery following the Great Recession.[21] Either of these phenomena would have affected Connecticut just as much as the comparison states. We conclude that Medicaid expansion in Connecticut offset what would have otherwise been an increased burden of uncompensated care because of these underlying dynamics.

It is important to note, however, that a simple interrupted time-series analysis that looked only at the flat trend in uncompensated care in Connecticut would conclude that the early expansion of Medicaid in 2010 had no effect on the amount of uncompensated care provided by hospitals. The trend in comparison states provides information needed to understand what would likely have happened in Connecticut in the absence of early Medicaid expansion.

REGRESSION We estimated multivariate difference-in-differences models to account for the possibility that other factors affecting uncompensated care, such as hospital size or local economic conditions, may have been changing differentially in Connecticut versus the other Northeastern states during this period. The models also included hospital and year fixed effects.

Consistent with Exhibits 2 and 3, the regression results in Exhibit 4 indicate that after expansion, Medicaid discharges increased significantly in Connecticut relative to the trend in the other states. When Medicaid discharges were measured as a share of total discharges, the regression-adjusted difference-in-differences model implies that Connecticut's early expansion increased the Medicaid share by 9.4 percentage points relative to the change in other states. This is an 85 percent increase relative to the baseline mean of 11.1 percent. We found a similar percentage increase for Medicaid dis-

EXHIBIT 4

Effects Of Medicaid Expansion In Connecticut Over Time, Compared To Changes In Comparison States

Dependent variable	Mean		Difference between periods	Difference-in-differences	
	Pre-expansion (2007-09)	Post-expansion (2011-13)		Unadjusted	Regression-adjusted
MEDICAID DISCHARGES					
As share of total				0.079***	0.094***
Connecticut	0.111	0.182	0.072		
Northeast	0.104	0.097	−0.007		
In levels				1,895***	2,814***
Connecticut	3,198	4,589	1,391		
Northeast	2,463	1,959	−504		
MEDICAID REVENUES					
As share of total				0.076***	0.070***
Connecticut	0.095	0.182	0.086		
Northeast	0.166	0.176	0.011		
In levels (millions of dollars)				158.3**	148.5***
Connecticut	135.8	356.6	220.9		
Northeast	307.9	370.5	62.5		
UNCOMPENSATED CARE					
As share of total expenses				−0.011***	−0.008
Connecticut	0.026	0.021	−0.005		
Northeast	0.027	0.033	0.006		
In levels (millions of dollars)				−5.1**	−3.8
Connecticut	13.9	11.4	−2.5		
Northeast	14.2	16.8	2.6		

SOURCE Authors' analysis of 2007–13 Medicare cost report data. **NOTES** The analysis sample included 1,744 observations from 434 hospitals in Connecticut and comparison states in the Northeast (Maine, New Hampshire, New York, Pennsylvania, Rhode Island, and Vermont). Observations from 2010 were omitted from the analysis because for most hospitals the 2010 fiscal year included both months before and months after Connecticut's implementation of the expansion of Medicaid. Results in levels represent the annual average per hospital number of Medicaid discharges; the annual average per hospital amount of Medicaid revenue in millions of dollars; and the annual average per hospital amount of uncompensated care in millions of dollars. All regressions were estimated using ordinary least squares and weighted by total discharges before expansion. Standard errors are clustered at the state level. To address the problem of clustering at the state level with only seven clusters, we estimated corrected p values by reestimating our main models using a data set of state-by-year means, following Donald SG, Lang K. Inference with difference-in-differences and other panel data. Rev Econ Stat. 2007;89(2):221–33. The regression-adjusted model included year and hospital fixed effects and controls for for-profit status, bed size, and county-level unemployment rate. **p < 0.05 ***p < 0.01

Uncompensated care may decline as a result of coverage expansions, but it will not go away.

charges measured in levels and for Medicaid revenues as a share of total revenues. When the dependent variable was measured in dollars, the regression-adjusted model implies that Medicaid revenues more than doubled: a relative increase of $148.5 million compared with a pre-expansion baseline of $135.8 million.

Turning to uncompensated care, the unadjusted difference-in-differences estimate implies that Connecticut's early Medicaid expansion reduced uncompensated care as a percentage of total hospital expenses by approximately 1 percentage point, or roughly one-third of the baseline mean (0.026). The point estimate from the regression-adjusted model was a slightly smaller and insignificant 0.8 percentage points. Measured in dollars, the results were similar, although the regression-adjusted estimate was marginally significant ($p = 0.11$).

ALTERNATIVE ANALYSES AND SENSITIVITY TESTS To test the sensitivity of our results, we conducted the analysis on alternative samples using alternative regression specifications. The results from these alternative models (Appendix Exhibit 5)[14] were not qualitatively different from those reported in Exhibit 4.

For our first robustness check, we limited the sample to hospitals with complete data for the entire study period. This reduced the sample to fifty-two hospitals and 364 hospital-year observations, but it did not change the results materially. The difference-in-differences estimates for this balanced sample imply that the early expansion of Medicaid increased the Medicaid share of discharges in Connecticut by 10 percentage points relative to comparison states and reduced uncompensated care as a percentage of total expenditures by 0.66 percentage points, which was marginally significant ($p = 0.10$).

Because all of the Connecticut hospitals in our sample were not for profit, we reestimated the regressions on a sample that excluded for-profit hospitals in the comparison states. Our results were robust to this change as well: We found that Medicaid discharges increased by 9 percentage

points, while uncompensated care fell by 0.81 percentage points.

Discussion

Connecticut was the first state to implement the ACA's Medicaid expansion by extending eligibility to childless adults who were not previously eligible for public insurance. The early expansion applied only to people with very low incomes (up to 56 percent of poverty). Nonetheless, it increased Medicaid enrollment by approximately 46,000 people and significantly reduced the number of uninsured adults.[10,12]

Our study investigated how this coverage expansion affected the provision of uncompensated care by hospitals in Connecticut. We found evidence that the volume of Medicaid discharges and revenue from Medicaid increased significantly. Uncompensated care in Connecticut did not increase, while it increased significantly in comparison states. This is consistent with preliminary evidence that since January 2014, hospitals in ACA expansion states have seen large increases in Medicaid patients.[6]

We also found that the implied reduction in the amount of uncompensated care in Connecticut relative to comparison states was much smaller than the increase in Medicaid revenue. One explanation for the difference in the size of these effects is that not all of the adults who gained Medicaid coverage in Connecticut were previously uninsured. In fact, Sommers and coauthors found that 40 percent of Connecticut's new Medicaid enrollees already had coverage.[12]

Bad debt generated by insured patients accounts for a significant portion of hospital uncompensated care. However, moving patients from private insurance to Medicaid should have a smaller effect on uncompensated care than extending coverage to the previously uninsured.

Because Medicaid payment rates are so much lower than those of private insurance, the substitution of public for private coverage tends to have a negative impact on total hospital revenues. We would expect crowd-out to be less of a factor for very poor adults, such as those who gained Medicaid coverage in Connecticut, than for the adults with slightly higher incomes who gained coverage in subsequent expansions that increased Medicaid eligibility to 138 percent of poverty. However, the degree of crowd-out that Sommers and coauthors found in Connecticut was greater than what has been projected for the ACA's national Medicaid expansion.[12,22] Going forward, the impact of health reform on hospitals will depend to an important degree on the extent to which increased public coverage displaces private insurance.

Conclusion

We close with three general observations about uncompensated care in a post-ACA world. First, uncompensated care may decline as a result of coverage expansions, but it will not go away. Current projections suggest that there will still be roughly thirty million uninsured people in the United States in 2025.[23] As long as there are uninsured patients, hospitals will continue to provide uncompensated care. Additional uncompensated care will be attributable to insured patients with unaffordable out-of-pocket expenses.

Second, policy makers have recently raised concerns about the level of charity care provided by not-for-profit hospitals,[24] and the regulatory environment is changing. These hospitals will face new and more stringent community benefit requirements under the ACA, beginning in 2016. The hospitals will be required to establish and publicize charity care policies and—before trying to collect patients' unpaid medical bills—to take steps to inform those patients that they could be eligible for charity care.

Third, it is reasonable to conclude that the reduction in uncompensated care caused by Connecticut's early Medicaid expansion represented a net gain for the state's hospitals. However, it is less clear what reductions in uncompensated care might mean for other actors in the system. Some advocates of health care reform have argued that reductions in uncompensated care provided by hospitals will translate into lower prices for private payers, which in turn will lead to lower premiums.[25] This argument is predicated on an assumption that hospitals engage in cost shifting. Although research on cost shifting is limited, the best evidence from rigorous empirical studies suggests that it is not a widespread phenomenon.[26]

Studies examining how hospitals respond to exogenous changes in public program reimbursement as well as to other financial shocks suggest a number of ways in which hospitals could use the savings from reduced uncompensated care. They could increase staffing levels,[27] investments in technology,[28] or holdings of financial assets.[29] Disentangling the effect of a reduction in uncompensated care from other changes in hospital finances brought about by the ACA is a challenging but important objective for future research. ∎

Results from this study were presented at the annual meeting of the Population Association of America, San Diego, California, May 1, 2015. Helen Levy received financial support from the National Institute on Aging (Grant No. NIA K01AG034232).

126

1 Ollove M. Hospitals lobby hard for Medicaid expansion. Stateline [blog on the Internet]. 2013 Apr 17 [cited 2015 Apr 30]. Available from: http://www.pewtrusts.org/en/research-and-analysis/blogs/stateline/2013/04/17/hospitals-lobby-hard-for-medicaid-expansion

2 Henry J. Kaiser Family Foundation. State health facts: status of state action on the Medicaid expansion decision [Internet]. Menlo Park (CA): KFF; 2015 Apr 29 [cited 2015 Apr 30]. Available from: http://kff.org/health-reform/state-indicator/state-activity-around-expanding-medicaid-under-the-affordable-care-act/

3 Graves JA. Medicaid expansion opt-outs and uncompensated care. N Engl J Med. 2012;367(25):2365-7.

4 Price CC, Eibner C. For states that opt out of Medicaid expansion: 3.6 million fewer insured and $8.4 billion less in federal payments. Health Aff (Millwood). 2013;32(6):1030-6.

5 Holahan J, Buettgens M, Dorn S. The cost of not expanding Medicaid [Internet]. Washington (DC): Kaiser Commission on Medicaid and the Uninsured; 2013 Jul 17 [cited 2015 Apr 30]. Available from: http://kff.org/medicaid/report/the-cost-of-not-expanding-medicaid/

6 DeLeire T, Joynt K, McDonald R. Impact of insurance expansion on hospital uncompensated care costs in 2014 [Internet]. Washington (DC): Department of Health and Human Services Office of the Assistant Secretary for Planning and Evaluation; 2014 Sep 24 [cited 2015 Apr 30]. (ASPE Issue Brief). Available from: http://aspe.hhs.gov/health/reports/2014/uncompensatedcare/ib_uncompensatedcare.pdf

7 Garthwaite C, Gross T, Notowidigdo MJ. Hospitals as insurers of last resort [Internet]. Unpublished paper. 2015 Jan [cited 2015 Apr 30]. Available from: http://faculty.wcas.northwestern.edu/noto/research/GGN_Hospitals%20as%20Insurers%20of%20Last%20Resort_jan2015.pdf

8 Arrieta A. The impact of the Massachusetts health care reform on unpaid medical bills. Inquiry. 2013;50(3):165-76.

9 Sommers BD, Arntson E, Kenney GM, Epstein AM. Lessons from early Medicaid expansions under health reform: interviews with Medicaid officials. Medicare Medicaid Res Rev. 2013;3(4).

10 State of Connecticut Department of Social Services. Section 1115 demonstration draft waiver application to the Centers for Medicare and Medicaid Services: Medicaid low-income adult coverage demonstration [Internet]. Hartford (CT): The Department; [cited 2015 Apr 30]. Available from: http://www.ct.gov/dss/lib/dss/pdfs/1115waivernewjune.pdf

11 Becker AL. Charter Oak health plan enrollment falls as premiums rise. CT Mirror [serial on the Internet]. 2011 Sep 9 [cited 2015 Apr 30]. Available from: http://ctmirror.org/2011/09/09/charter-oak-health-plan-enrollment-falls-premiums-rise/

12 Sommers BD, Kenney GM, Epstein AM. New evidence on the Affordable Care Act: coverage impacts of early Medicaid expansions. Health Aff (Millwood). 2014;33(1):78-87.

13 American Hospital Association. Uncompensated hospital care cost fact sheet [Internet]. Chicago (IL): AHA; 2014 Jan [cited 2015 May 1]. Available from: http://www.aha.org/content/14/14uncompensatedcare.pdf

14 To access the Appendix, click on the Appendix link in the box to the right of the article online.

15 Kane NM, Magnus SA. The Medicare cost report and the limits of hospital accountability: improving financial accounting data. J Health Polit Policy Law. 2001;26(1):81-105.

16 American Hospital Association. Fast facts on US hospitals [Internet]. Chicago (IL): AHA; [updated 2015 Jan; cited 2015 May 1]. Available from: http://www.aha.org/research/rc/stat-studies/fast-facts.shtml

17 Government Accountability Office. Nonprofit, for-profit, and government hospitals: uncompensated care and other community benefits [Internet]. Washington (DC): GAO; 2005 May 26 [cited 2015 May 1]. (Report No. GAO-05-743T). Available from: http://www.gao.gov/new.items/d05743t.pdf

18 Baicker K, Taubman S, Allen H, Bernstein M, Gruber J, Newhouse J, et al. The Oregon experiment—effect of Medicaid on clinical outcomes. N Engl J Med. 2013;368(18):1713-22.

19 Hancock J. More high-deductible plan members can't pay hospital bills. Kaiser Health News [serial on the Internet]. 2013 Aug 12 [cited 2015 May 1]. Available from: http://kaiserhealthnews.org/news/more-high-deductible-plan-members-cant-pay-hospital-bills/

20 Rowe J. Uncompensated care an ominous trend. Healthcare Finance [serial on the Internet]. 2011 Jun 2 [cited 2015 May 1]. Available from: http://www.healthcarefinance-news.com/news/uncompensated-care-ominous-trend

21 Karash JA. Bad debt. The rising tide of uncompensated care. Hosp Health Netw. 2010;84(2):11.

22 Buettgens M. Health Insurance Policy Simulation Model (HIPSM) methodology documentation [Internet]. Washington (DC): Urban Institute; 2011 Dec 21 [cited 2015 May 1]. (Research Report). Available from: http://www.urban.org/research/publication/health-insurance-policy-simulation-model-hipsm-methodology-documentation

23 Congressional Budget Office. Insurance coverage provisions of the Affordable Care Act—CBO's April 2014 baseline [Internet]. Washington (DC): CBO; [cited 2015 May 1]. Available from: https://www.cbo.gov/sites/default/files/cbofiles/attachments/43900-2014-04-ACAtables2.pdf

24 Grassley C. Letter to Mosaic Life Care [Internet]. Washington (DC): Senate Committee on the Judiary; 2015 Jan 16 [cited 2015 May 1]. Available from: http://www.propublica.org/documents/item/1503959-grassley-letter-2015-01-16-ceg-to-mosaic.html

25 Stoll K, Bailey K. Hidden health tax: Americans pay a premium [Internet]. Washington (DC): Families USA; 2009 May [cited 2015 May 1]. Available from: http://familiesusa.org/sites/default/files/product_documents/hidden-health-tax.pdf

26 Frakt AB. How much do hospitals cost shift? A review of the evidence. Milbank Q. 2011;89(1):90-130.

27 White C, Wu VY. How do hospitals cope with sustained slow growth in Medicare prices? Health Serv Res. 2014;49(1):11-31.

28 Dranove D, Garthwaite C, Ody C. How do hospitals respond to negative financial shocks? The impact of the 2008 stock market crash [Internet]. Cambridge (MA): National Bureau of Economic Research; 2013 Feb [cited 2015 May 1]. (NBER Working Paper No. 18853). Available from: http://www.nber.org/papers/w18853

29 Duggan MG. Hospital ownership and public medical spending. Q J Econ. 2000;115(4):1343-73.

127

HealthAffairs

At the Intersection of Health, Health Care and Policy

Cite this article as:
Randall D. Cebul, Thomas E. Love, Douglas Einstadter, Alice S. Petrulis and John R.
Corlett
MetroHealth Care Plus: Effects Of A Prepared Safety Net On Quality Of Care In A
Medicaid Expansion Population
Health Affairs, 34, no.7 (2015):1121-1130

doi: 10.1377/hlthaff.2014.1380

The online version of this article, along with updated information and services, is
available at:
http://content.healthaffairs.org/content/34/7/1121.full.html

For Reprints, Links & Permissions:
http://healthaffairs.org/1340_reprints.php

E-mail Alerts : http://content.healthaffairs.org/subscriptions/etoc.dtl

To Subscribe: http://content.healthaffairs.org/subscriptions/online.shtml

Health Affairs is published monthly by Project HOPE at 7500 Old Georgetown Road, Suite 600,
Bethesda, MD 20814-6133. Copyright © 2015 by Project HOPE - The People-to-People Health
Foundation. As provided by United States copyright law (Title 17, U.S. Code), no part of *Health
Affairs* may be reproduced, displayed, or transmitted in any form or by any means, electronic or
mechanical, including photocopying or by information storage or retrieval systems, without prior
written permission from the Publisher. All rights reserved.

Not for commercial use or unauthorized distribution

Downloaded from content.healthaffairs.org by *Health Affairs* on September 23, 2015
by guest

MEDICAID & PRIMARY CARE

By Randall D. Cebul, Thomas E. Love, Douglas Einstadter, Alice S. Petrulis, and John R. Corlett

MetroHealth Care Plus: Effects Of A Prepared Safety Net On Quality Of Care In A Medicaid Expansion Population

DOI: 10.1377/hlthaff.2014.1380
HEALTH AFFAIRS 34,
NO. 7 (2015): 1121-1130
©2015 Project HOPE—
The People-to-People Health
Foundation, Inc.

ABSTRACT Studies of Medicaid expansion have produced conflicting results about whether the expansion is having a positive impact on health and the cost and efficiency of care delivery. To explore the issue further, we examined MetroHealth Care Plus, a Centers for Medicare and Medicaid Services (CMS) waiver program in Ohio composed of three safety-net organizations that enrolled 28,295 uninsured poor patients in closed-panel care during 2013. All participating organizations used electronic health records and patient-centered medical homes, publicly reported performance in a regional health improvement collaborative, and accepted a budget-neutral cap approved by CMS. We compared changes between 2012 and 2013 in achieving quality standards for diabetes and hypertension among 3,437 MetroHealth Care Plus enrollees to changes among 1,150 patients with the same conditions who remained uninsured in both years. Compared to continuously uninsured patients with diabetes, MetroHealth Care Plus enrollees with diabetes improved significantly more on composite standards of care and intermediate outcomes. Among enrollees with hypertension, blood pressure control improvements were insignificantly larger than those in the continuously uninsured group with hypertension. Across all 28,295 enrollees, 2013 total costs of care were 28.7 percent below the budget cap, providing cause for optimism that a prepared safety net can meet the challenges of Medicaid expansion.

Randall D. Cebul (rdc@case.edu) is president of the Better Health Partnership, a professor in the Departments of Medicine and of Epidemiology and Biostatistics at Case Western Reserve University, and director of the Case Western Reserve University Center for Health Care Research and Policy at MetroHealth Medical Center, all in Cleveland, Ohio.

Thomas E. Love is data director of the Better Heath Partnership and a professor in the Departments of Medicine and of Epidemiology and Biostatistics at Case Western Reserve University and at the Case Western Reserve University Center for Health Care Research and Policy at MetroHealth Medical Center.

Douglas Einstadter is a professor in the Departments of Medicine and of Epidemiology and Biostatistics at Case Western Reserve University and at the Case Western Reserve University Center for Health Care Research and Policy at MetroHealth Medical Center.

Alice S. Petrulis is a professor in the Department of Medicine at Case Western Reserve University.

John R. Corlett was vice president for government relations and community affairs at the MetroHealth System when this research was conducted. He is now president and executive director of the Center for Community Solutions, in Cleveland.

As Medicaid expansion continues under Affordable Care Act (ACA) provisions, debate continues about its likely impact on health and on the cost and efficiency of care delivery. Fueling the debate are conflicting results from studies using various methods, including recent studies emphasizing coverage expansion.[1-3]

For example, in 2012 Benjamin Sommers and coauthors documented favorable changes in population-level access to care, self-reported health status, and all-cause mortality in three states where Medicaid coverage had expanded since 2000, compared to three contiguous states with no expansion.[1] And in 2013 Katherine Baicker and colleagues reported on Oregon's 2008 Medicaid expansion that enabled poor uninsured winners of a lottery to apply for Medicaid while lottery losers were left uninsured.[2] After two years, Oregon's newly insured Medicaid patients had no significant differences in physical health and no differences in self-reported use of emergency department (ED) services, compared to lottery losers. Follow-up administrative data from Portland-area hospitals documented 40 percent higher ED use—including "preventable" use—among patients in the expansion group,[3] compared to the uninsured control group.

Before Ohio approved its ACA Medicaid expansion in October 2013, the state had received a waiver enabling safety-net organizations in its largest county—Cuyahoga—to provide closed-panel care coverage under a budget-neutral cap approved by the Centers for Medicare and Medicaid Services (CMS). In the MetroHealth Care Plus program, the county-owned MetroHealth System and two of the county's federally qualified health centers enrolled patients with family incomes at or below 133 percent of the federal poverty level.

The three organizations used the same electronic health record (EHR) system, which enabled them to exchange health information. All but two of the organizations' eighteen primary care practice sites had received recognition as level 3 patient-centered medical homes from the National Committee for Quality Assurance; had used nurses for care coordination; and participated in a regional health improvement collaborative, Better Health Partnership.

Better Health uses EHRs to measure and publicly report achievement on quality of care for chronic conditions, including diabetes and hypertension. This study used Better Health's data to compare changes in quality measures for these two conditions among established patients of the MetroHealth System who enrolled in MetroHealth Care Plus to changes among patients with the same conditions who remained uninsured.

Study Data And Methods

THE INTERVENTION: METROHEALTH CARE PLUS

▶ WAIVER CONDITIONS: In February 2013 CMS approved an Ohio Medicaid application for a waiver, which allowed the MetroHealth System to proceed with a coverage expansion program based in a safety-net institution.[4] Called MetroHealth Care Plus, the program provided coverage to uninsured adults ages 18–64 who had family incomes at or below 133 percent of poverty, met US citizenship or legal immigrant requirements, resided in Cuyahoga County, and were not otherwise eligible for Medicaid benefits.

MetroHealth Care Plus patients received benefits through a defined provider network that consisted of the county-owned MetroHealth System and community provider partners, including two federally qualified health centers and the region's community mental health centers. The waiver supported enrollment of up to 30,000 county residents under an allowed budget-neutral expenditure cap per member

month approved by CMS.

▶ COVERAGE BENEFITS: The waiver allowed MetroHealth Care Plus to offer benefits for many services that were previously unavailable under the long-standing income-based rating methods used to determine health benefits and costs for uninsured county residents. Under the waiver program, no copayments were required for any service. These previously unavailable services included routine dental care, durable medical equipment, emergency and nonemergency medical transportation, short-term nursing facility services, home health services, selected additional substance abuse services, and services at the federally qualified health centers that were partners in the waiver program.

▶ ACTUARIAL ANALYSES FOR RATE SETTING: To prepare the waiver application, the MetroHealth System and Ohio Medicaid employed an independent actuarial firm to analyze utilization and cost data for the MetroHealth System's relevant uninsured population that were augmented by data from Medicaid. Per member month rates were estimated that accounted for utilization and unit costs for each service, including benefits for the new services described above and required out-of-network reimbursements; adjustments for services that may have been incurred but not reported; and projected trends with and without the waiver.

The actuarial methods were submitted by the state and accepted by CMS, and the associated per member month rates were modified to reflect an allowable federal budget-neutral cap on expenditures.[4] Using these methods, the expenditure cap was set at an average of $582.41 per enrollee per month. If, at the end of the demonstration period, the cumulative expenditure cap had been exceeded, excess federal funds would have been required to be returned to CMS.[4]

▶ RECRUITMENT AND ENROLLMENT: Marketing of the waiver program was undertaken through a variety of publicity and community outreach activities to inform relevant agencies and potentially eligible patient populations. In addition to publicity in the media to reach county residents, marketing materials were distributed to community groups and public organizations, and program representatives attended meetings to answer questions.

Two general methods of enrollment were employed, as called for in the terms and conditions that the State of Ohio imposed on MetroHealth Care Plus. The first method, applications by individuals at their own initiative, was facilitated by community agencies and the patients' health care providers. Uninsured patients who were hospitalized during the enrollment period and determined to be eligible for MetroHealth Care

Plus were invited to enroll. The second approach enabled MetroHealth Care Plus to automatically enroll patients who were determined to be eligible effective February 5, 2013, based on their current enrollment in the MetroHealth System's income-based rating program to determine health benefits for the poor.

New enrollees were given educational materials that covered a variety of topics. The materials informed enrollees how to maximize the use of their new medical and pharmaceutical benefit coverage, how to rely on primary care providers, how to present their new identification cards when seeking care, and how to adhere to providers' care instructions.

▶ SITES AND CARE DELIVERY: MetroHealth Care Plus enrollees accessed care coordination services through primary care–based patient-centered medical home sites within the Metro-Health System (which had twelve sites) or one of the two federally qualified health centers (which together had six sites). As noted above, all but two of the eighteen sites had received recognition as level 3 patient-centered medical homes from the National Committee for Quality Assurance before the waiver program commenced and used EHRs from the same vendor (EpicCare, in Verona, Wisconsin), which enables vendor-specific health information exchange (described elsewhere).[5]

Enrolled patients who had established relationships with primary care providers maintained them. Other patients were encouraged at enrollment to select a patient-centered medical home and primary care provider in the network. Because the demonstration provided support for nurse care coordinators, these caregivers were able to use the EHR system to contact patients, monitor them, and provide problem-centered care plans.

Twice yearly all care sites measured and publicly reported their adult patients' achievement on diabetes and hypertension standards as part of Better Health, one of sixteen collaboratives nationwide supported by the Robert Wood Johnson Foundation's Aligning Forces for Quality initiative.[6]

The MetroHealth System's 732-bed county-owned hospital, the region's principal safety-net provider, served as the preferred site for inpatient care and referral outpatient care for all MetroHealth Care Plus enrollees. Other area hospitals entered into out-of-network payment arrangements with MetroHealth Care Plus, including necessary ED services. The program's third-party administrator provided claims reports, daily enrollment file exchange with MetroHealth Care Plus, and communications with MetroHealth Care Plus's medical director (Alice Petrulis, one of the authors).

STUDY GOALS AND PATIENT ELIGIBILITY In our primary analyses, we examined changes in care and intermediate outcome measures among a subset of MetroHealth Care Plus enrollees with diabetes, hypertension, or both in 2013 who were uninsured and who were established patient-centered medical home patients who received care within the MetroHealth System during 2012. We used prespecified eligibility and quality criteria established by Better Health.[7]

Patients with diabetes were eligible for inclusion in our study population if they were ages 18–63 in 2012 and made at least two visits to the same practice in both 2012 and 2013.[8] Patients with hypertension (defined by *International Classification of Diseases*, Ninth Revision [ICD9], codes 401–405.9 on the EHR problem list) were eligible for inclusion in our study if they were ages 18–63 in 2012 and made at least two visits to the same practice over the two-year period, including at least one visit in each measurement year.[9] We compared 2012 to 2013 changes for MetroHealth Care Plus enrollees who met the diabetes and hypertension criteria to changes among continuously uninsured patients who met the same eligibility criteria but were not enrolled in the MetroHealth Care Plus program.

In secondary analyses, to detect potential declines in performance on quality measures that were not publicly reported by Better Health, we tested for analogous differences-in-changes (differences-in-differences) in the provision of vaccinations, cancer screening, and depression screening or monitoring. We also report 2013 total costs of care (a summary of all paid claims for services rendered during the program) compared to the CMS-approved budget-neutral cap.

ENDPOINTS, MEASURES, AND DATA SOURCES The primary study endpoints were quality of care and intermediate clinical outcomes for patients with documented diabetes, hypertension, or both, as required for Better Health public reporting.[7] All data were obtained from the EHR. As described elsewhere,[10] composite standards for diabetes care and clinical outcomes have been reported twice yearly since 2008.

The four measures in the diabetes care composite standard are checking the patient's hemoglobin A1c, monitoring or managing renal dysfunction using a urine microalbumin screen or prescribing an angiotensin-converting enzyme (ACE) inhibitor or angiotensin receptor blocker (ARB), performing a dilated eye examination, and administering a pneumococcal vaccination. Except for the vaccination, measured as "ever received," all measures pertain to the relevant twelve-month interval, which for this study was either 2012 or 2013.

13+

Percentage points
MetroHealth Care Plus patients with diabetes improved over 13 percentage points more on the diabetes composite standard than did members of the continuously uninsured group.

The diabetes care composite standard is reported as an "all or nothing" patient-level standard. In other words, each patient-centered medical home site receives credit for the percentage of its patients who met the criteria for all four of the measures in the relevant twelve-month period.[10]

The diabetes outcome composite standard is based on the following five measures: good Hb A1c control (<8 percent), good blood pressure control (<140/90 mmHg),[11,12] good control of low-density lipoprotein (LDL) cholesterol (<100 mg/dl or the prescription of a statin), good weight control (body mass index <30), and nonsmoking status. Successful achievement of the patient-level outcome composite standard requires that at least four of the five standards are met.[10]

For patients with hypertension, our all-or-nothing composite care standard consisted of checking blood pressure at every visit and annually measuring serum creatinine and LDL cholesterol.[9,13] As above, good blood pressure control was defined as less than 140/90 mmHg.[9]

To detect potential declines in performance on quality measures that were not publicly reported, possibly as a result of paying less attention to the nonreported standards than to the reported ones, we examined as secondary clinical endpoints the timely receipt of selected preventive services not included in Better Health's publicly reported care standards. These preventive services included providing a tetanus booster for patients ages 18–64 if they had not received one in the previous ten years, mammography for women ages 50–64 if they had not received a mammogram during the previous two years, a Pap test for women ages 21–64 if they had not received one within the previous three years, and colon cancer screening for people ages 50–64 if they had not completed a fecal occult blood test in the previous year or had sigmoidoscopy within the previous five years or a colonoscopy within the previous ten years.

In addition, in 2012 MetroHealth established a protocol for another preventive service: yearly screening for depression and monitoring via the Patient Health Questionnaire (PHQ)[14] for those with a depression diagnosis (ICD-9 codes 296.2–296.39, 300.4, or 311 on the EHR problem list).

Total costs of care of MetroHealth Care Plus enrollees were compared to the budget-neutral expenditure cap, since there were no cost data available among the continuously uninsured comparison group for their care at unaffiliated health care organizations. We used claims paid through MetroHealth Care Plus's third-party administrator to determine utilization rates per 1,000 enrollees per year for selected service categories and total costs of care for all patients across all sites for the period February 5–December 31, 2013.

Costs were summarized per member month across all enrollees and compared to the CMS-approved budget-neutral cap. We used the duration of each person's enrollment to calculate the number of member months at the patient level. Total per member month costs were calculated by dividing the sum of all member months by the total cost associated with adjudicated claims from the beginning of the waiver program through mid-2014.

STATISTICAL ANALYSIS Our difference-in-changes estimates[15] compared 2012-to-2013 changes for patients enrolled in MetroHealth Care Plus who met the diabetes and hypertension criteria to changes over the same period for those who were continuously uninsured. We accounted for random patient effects via linear mixed-effect models, which we fit using R, version 3.1.2. As an example, for the diabetes outcome composite standard, the change from 2012 to 2013 in MetroHealth Care Plus was 4.7 percentage points, while the same change in the continuously uninsured was −3.7 percentage points, making the difference-in-changes 8.4 percentage points. We used heteroskedasticity-consistent sandwich estimates of the variance-covariance matrix to formulate confidence intervals.[16,17]

The MetroHealth System's Human Privacy Board approved this investigation's data collection and submission protocols.

LIMITATIONS Several limitations of this investigation should be noted. The 3,437 eligible MetroHealth Care Plus enrollees in this study accounted for over 44 percent of all MetroHealth Care Plus enrollees with diabetes, hypertension, or both, but for only 12.1 percent of the total MetroHealth Care Plus enrollment of 28,295 patients (online Appendix Exhibits B and C).[18] Both MetroHealth Care Plus enrollees and the comparison group were adults with documented hypertension, diabetes, or both in both 2012 and 2013 and had sufficient continuity of primary care within the MetroHealth System to be eligible for Better Health's public reporting.[7,10] These patients had highly prevalent and important chronic conditions, which enabled us to identify similar patients who were continuously uninsured. However, our differences-in-changes should not be generalized to other MetroHealth Care Plus enrollees or patients who lack continuity of care.

Most patients in both study groups had established relationships with their primary providers. Our requirement for continuous primary care meant that patients in the study were more likely to have better outcomes than those with fragmented care or poor access to care.[19-21] A recent investigation of the Oregon experiment documented poorer patient-reported outcomes among those who reported confusion about coverage or perceived barriers to access, and better outcomes among those who reported multiple health care interactions, continuity of care, and easier patient-provider interaction.[22]

In our preliminary examination of trends in use (Appendix Exhibit L),[18] we found that hospitalization rates per 1,000 enrollees per year were highest in the earliest months of the waiver. In contrast, utilization rates of other service categories reported here (the ED and outpatient and dental services) peaked during the second or third month. We believe that patterns of higher use of the ED and hospital in early months likely reflected voluntary enrollment of eligible patients at the time of their hospitalizations, previous unmet need, and lack of familiarity with the primary care–centered focus of MetroHealth Care Plus. The latter factor may have been especially relevant among people who were automatically enrolled based on their then-current enrollment in the MetroHealth System's income-based rating system for health benefits.

The declines in use of all reported service categories after March or April are encouraging. However, the fact that people were enrolled in MetroHealth Care Plus for only a short time (eleven months maximum, nine months median) limits the inferences that can be drawn from our results and their generalizability to similar programs elsewhere.

The favorable results of our cost-related analyses likewise are limited by the absence of analogous costs for the continuously uninsured. In addition, the magnitude of the CMS-approved expenditure cap in MetroHealth Care Plus was mostly a reflection of regional service experience among the uninsured and Ohio Medicaid patient populations. This limited our ability to make broad inferences about what savings are likely to accrue in Medicaid expansions for other populations.

Nonetheless, these data describe total costs of care across a large countywide waiver population, and those costs were 28.7 percent lower and more than $41 million less than allowable under the contract with CMS.

Study Results

ENROLLMENT AND BASELINE CHARACTERISTICS Between February 5 and December 31, 2013, 28,295 uninsured adults enrolled in Metro-Health Care Plus. Over 75 percent (21,484) of these patients enrolled during the first four months of the program, and the median duration of enrollment was nine months, as noted above (Appendix Exhibit A shows the trajectory of enrollment).[18] Of the total, 9,205 (33 percent) were automatically enrolled based on their then-current enrollment in the MetroHealth System's income-based rating program, while 19,090 (67 percent) enrolled on their own initiative.

Altogether, there were 3,437 MetroHealth Care Plus patients who met diabetes, hypertension, or both criteria for inclusion in the study population (12.1 percent of the entire Metro-Health Care Plus enrollment population) and 1,150 continuously uninsured patients who received care within the MetroHealth System and who met Better Health's criteria for public reporting for diabetes, hypertension, or both during both 2012 and 2013 (Exhibit 1).

Patients in the MetroHealth Care Plus diabetes and hypertension subset represented 44.4 percent of all MetroHealth Care Plus patients with one or both of these conditions at the end of 2013 and were demographically similar to those who enrolled but did not meet Better Health's criteria for public reporting of diabetes, hypertension, or both (Appendix Exhibits B and C).[18]

At baseline, compared to the continuously un-

EXHIBIT 1

Baseline Characteristics Of Patients In The MetroHealth Care Plus (MHCP) And Continuously Uninsured Study Groups

Characteristic	MHCP (N = 3,437)	Uninsured (N = 1,150)	Difference*
SOCIODEMOGRAPHIC CHARACTERISTICS (ALL PATIENTS)			
Mean age (years)	50.9	52.2	−1.4**
Female	59.9%	63.5%	−3.5**
Race			**
White	34.6%	40.9%	−6.3
African American	56.9	45.9	11.0
Other	8.4	13.2	−4.8
Cleveland resident	59.1%	55.7%	3.4**
Estimated median income ($1,000s)	$36.0	$37.9	−$1.9**
Estimated high school graduates	79.9%	80.0%	−0.1
CLINICAL CHARACTERISTICS (ALL PATIENTS)			
EHR-documented depression diagnosis	29.9%	26.3%	3.6**
Good blood pressure control (<140/90 mmHg)	55.8	58.8	−3.0
Body mass index <30	37.3	38.0	−0.7
Not smoking	64.8	70.6	−5.8**
PREVENTIVE SERVICES RECEIVED (ELIGIBLE PATIENTS ONLY)			
Tetanus shot	91.7%	91.6%	0.1
Mammography[b]	79.1	75.7	3.5
Colon cancer screening[b]	71.2	67.8	3.4
Pap test[b]	76.0	75.0	1.0
Body mass index check	99.7	99.7	0.1

SOURCE Authors' analysis of data from Better Health Partnership and the MetroHealth System. **NOTES** Preventive services are described in more detail in the text. EHR is electronic health record. *Years, dollars, or percentage points. [b]Not all patients were eligible for this measure. **p < 0.05

insured, MetroHealth Care Plus patients in the study group had a number of features associated with lower achievement on quality standards, especially those requiring better adherence to medical recommendations or larger out-of-pocket expenses for health care services. In particular, MetroHealth Care Plus enrollees were more likely to be nonwhite (65.4 percent versus 59.1 percent), to live in the city of Cleveland (59.1 percent versus 55.7 percent) and in poorer neighborhoods (estimated median income $36,000 versus $37,900), to have an EHR-documented depression diagnosis (29.9 percent versus 26.3 percent), and to be a current smoker (35.2 percent versus 29.4 percent). In 2012 the two groups had similar rates of receipt of the preventive services in our study that were not publicly reported by Better Health.

Appendix Exhibits D and E compare the clinical characteristics of the study groups by medical condition.[18] Of patients with diabetes, those in MetroHealth Care Plus were significantly less likely than those in the continuously uninsured group to achieve our composite diabetes outcome standard in 2012 (32.9 percent versus 40.1 percent). MetroHealth Care Plus enrollees were less likely than members of the continuously uninsured group to achieve eight of the nine individual diabetes standards. However, there were no significant differences between the groups on the individual outcome mea-

sures, care measures, or diabetes care composite standard.[18]

Among patients with hypertension, rates of good blood pressure control were similar in the two groups. Rates of individual quality care measures were all over 90 percent, and they were virtually identical in the two groups.[18]

CHANGES IN MEASURES FOR DIABETES AND HYPERTENSION MetroHealth Care Plus patients with diabetes improved over 13 percentage points (95% confidence interval: 4.3, 22.1) more on the composite standard for diabetes care than did members of the continuously uninsured group (Exhibit 2). The difference between the two groups in the change in the proportion of patients receiving dilated eye examinations was the largest contributor to the significant difference between them in the all-or-nothing composite standard.

Rates of pneumococcal vaccinations also improved significantly among MetroHealth Care Plus enrollees who met the diabetes criteria, but not significantly more than among the continuously uninsured (Exhibit 2). Both groups had high baseline rates of hemoglobin A1c testing and testing for or treatment of kidney dysfunction (microalbumin screen or prescription of an ACE inhibitor or an ARB), and there were no significant differences-in-changes between the groups (details are provided in Appendix Exhibits F–H).[18]

MetroHealth Care Plus patients with diabetes improved more on the composite diabetes outcome standard (difference-in-changes: 8.4 percentage points; 95% CI: 1.9, 14.9) than did the continuously uninsured comparison group (Exhibit 3). Significantly more MetroHealth Care Plus patients met the good blood pressure target than did patients who were continuously uninsured (difference-in-changes: 7.9 percentage points; 95% CI: 0.1, 15.7). There were no significant differences-in-changes between the two groups in the other standards.

MetroHealth Care Plus patients with hypertension showed significant improvement in rates of good blood pressure control during the waiver year. However, parallel improvements among the continuously uninsured made the difference-in-changes not significant (2.8 percentage points; 95% CI: -1.6, 7.1; Exhibit 4). In secondary analyses, we found that MetroHealth Care Plus patients with hypertension were more likely to have been prescribed at least one antihypertensive medication (difference-in-changes: 1.9 percentage points; 95% CI: 0.2, 3.5).

Both groups had a high rate of achievement of care standards for hypertension at baseline. Compared to continuously uninsured patients, MetroHealth Care Plus patients showed more

---

EXHIBIT 2

Diabetes Care For Patients In The MetroHealth Care Plus (MHCP) And Continuously Uninsured Study Groups, 2012–13

Measure	2012	2013	Change over time[a]	Difference-in-changes[a]
Diabetes care composite				
MHCP	50.9%	59.7%	8.8**	13.2**
Uninsured	53.2	48.8	−4.4	
Hemoglobin A1c checked				
MHCP	99.1	99.7	0.6	0.3
Uninsured	99.7	100.0	0.3	
Microalbumin screen or prescription of ACE inhibitor or ARB				
MHCP	97.4	98.4	1.0	0.0
Uninsured	98.3	99.3	1.0	
Dilated eye examination				
MHCP	55.6	63.1	7.6**	13.3**
Uninsured	57.9	52.2	−5.7	
Pneumococcal vaccination				
MHCP	91.2	94.2	3.0**	1.7
Uninsured	91.3	92.6	1.4	

SOURCE Authors' analysis of data from Better Health Partnership and the MetroHealth System. **NOTES** There were 963 patients in the MHCP group and 297 in the uninsured group. Difference-in-changes are the differences between the two groups' changes over time. The diabetes composite measure consists of the four other measures, described in more detail in the text. Compliance with the composite measure is defined as compliance with all four of the measures. ACE is angiotensin-converting enzyme. ARB is angiotensin receptor blocker. [a]Percentage points. **$p < 0.05$

improvement in having checks of serum creatinine to test kidney function (difference-in-changes: 0.8 percentage point; 95% CI: 0.2, 1.3). There were no significant differences between the groups on the other measures (Appendix Exhibits H and I).[18]

CHANGES IN SECONDARY CLINICAL MEASURES We found no significant differences-in-changes between the two groups in rates of appropriate immunizations for tetanus and screenings for breast, colorectal, and cervical cancer (Appendix Exhibits J and K).[18] By contrast, MetroHealth Care Plus enrollees showed higher rates of screening or monitoring for depression using the PHQ, compared to the uninsured group (difference-in-changes: 4.9 percentage points; 95% CI: 1.6, 8.2). However, both groups showed large increases from 2012 to 2013.

USE AND TOTAL COSTS OF CARE Appendix Exhibit L summarizes trends in use of selected categories of service in rates per 1,000 enrollees per year.[18] Hospitalization rates declined from 62.8 per 1,000 enrollees per year in February to 44.4 in December. Use of other services (including outpatient and dental services and ED use) increased during the first few months before leveling off or declining thereafter.

Total costs of care for MetroHealth Care Plus enrollees were compared to the CMS-approved budget-neutral cap on a per member-month basis. There were 250,514 eligible member-months among the 28,295 MetroHealth Care Plus enrollees during the waiver program. As of June 2014— when sufficient time had elapsed for submission and adjudication of claims for 2013 services— total per member-month costs for MetroHealth Care Plus patients averaged $415.05, or $167.36 (28.7 percent) lower than the $582.41 budget-neutral cap.

The CMS-allowed expenditure cap for all eligible enrollees was $145 million. Actual expenditures for services provided were $104 million, or approximately $41 million lower than what CMS had allowed.[4]

Discussion

The Oregon experiment[3] has generated considerable debate about Medicaid expansion among policy makers and in the popular press.[23-25] Both it and the MetroHealth Care Plus waiver were intended to provide estimates of the impact of expanding health coverage on measures of physical health. However, the designs and results of the two interventions differed substantially.

The MetroHealth Care Plus intervention focused on contemporary delivery system innovations among safety-net organizations that accepted closed-panel care and a federally im-

EXHIBIT 3

Outcomes For Patients With Diabetes In The MetroHealth Care Plus (MHCP) And Continuously Uninsured Study Groups, 2012–13

Outcome	2012	2013	Change over time[a]	Difference-in-changes[a]
Diabetes outcomes composite measure				
MHCP	32.9%	37.6%	4.7**	8.4**
Uninsured	40.1	36.4		
Hemoglobin A1c <8%				
MHCP	61.2	61.2	0.0	2.4
Uninsured	63.0	60.6	−2.4	
Good blood pressure control (<140/90 mmHg)				
MHCP	58.4	63.2	4.9**	7.9**
Uninsured	64.7	61.6	−3.0	
LDL <100 mg/dl or statin prescription				
MHCP	85.5	88.7	3.2	−0.8
Uninsured	84.9	88.9	4.0	
Body mass index <30				
MHCP	29.6	30.6	1.0	1.4
Uninsured	34.0	33.7	−0.3	
Documented as not smoking				
MHCP	69.3	71.0	1.8	0.8
Uninsured	74.4	75.4	1.0	

SOURCE Authors' analysis of data from Better Health Partnership and the MetroHealth System. **NOTES** There were 963 patients in the MHCP group and 297 in the uninsured group. Difference-in-changes are the differences between the two groups' changes over time. The diabetes outcomes composite measure consists of the five outcomes below it. Achieving the composite outcome is defined as achieving at least four of the five included outcomes. LDL is low-density lipoprotein cholesterol. [a]Percentage points. **p < 0.05

posed expenditure cap. All of the care sites in the MetroHealth Care Plus program participated in Better Health, an EHR-catalyzed regional health improvement collaborative that publicly reported performance. This helped accelerate the development of relevant infrastructure for quality improvement and provided the patient-level data needed to examine changes in quality across both newly covered and continuously uninsured patients.

By contrast, the Oregon experiment almost exclusively focused on coverage expansion, with little attention paid to care delivery models, providers' interest in patient enrollment, or the providers' experience with improving care quality.[3] MetroHealth Care Plus enrollment was driven by safety-net organizations eager to reduce barriers to the delivery of high-quality care and was brisk, which resulted in a rapid reduction in the region's uninsured population.[26] In contrast, participation in the Oregon experiment was limited, and people were slow to enroll.[27]

Despite having adverse baseline characteristics compared to the continuously uninsured[28] and only nine months' average enrollment, MetroHealth Care Plus enrollees had significantly better improvements in diabetes care and outcomes than the improvements in the continu-

MEDICAID & PRIMARY CARE

EXHIBIT 4

Care For Patients With High Blood Pressure In The MetroHealth Care Plus (MHCP) And Continuously Uninsured Study Groups, 2012–13

Measure	2012	2013	Change over time[a]	Difference-in-changes[a]
Good blood pressure (<140/90 mmHg)				
MHCP	54.5%	58.4%	3.9**	2.8
Uninsured	57.6	58.7	1.1	
High blood pressure care composite measure				
MHCP	94.1	95.9	1.8**	0.6
Uninsured	94.6	95.9	1.2	
Blood pressure check				
MHCP	100	100	0.0	0.0
Uninsured	100	100	0.0	
Serum creatinine check				
MHCP	99.1	99.9	0.8**	0.8**
Uninsured	99.5	99.5	0.0	
LDL cholesterol check				
MHCP	94.4	96.0	1.6**	0.4
Uninsured	94.8	96.1	1.2	
Prescription of antihypertensive medication[b]				
MHCP	94.3	94.9	0.5	1.9**
Uninsured	94.2	92.9	−1.3	

SOURCE Authors' analysis of data from Better Health Partnership and the MetroHealth System. **NOTES** There were 3,185 patients in the MHCP group and 1,063 patients in the uninsured group. Difference-in-changes are the differences between the two groups' changes over time. The high blood pressure care composite measure consists of checks of blood pressure, serum creatinine, and LDL cholesterol. Compliance with the composite measure is defined as compliance with all three standards. LDL is low-density lipoprotein cholesterol. [a]Percentage points. [b]Antihypertensive medications include angiotensin-converting enzyme inhibitors, angiotensin receptor blockers, diuretics, calcium channel blockers, beta-blockers, alpha-1 blockers, centrally acting alpha-2 agonists, and vasodilators. **$p < 0.05$

ously uninsured group. Changes in care were dominated by improvements in dilated eye examinations, with lesser improvements in care standards that showed high levels of achievement (over 90 percent) at baseline for both study groups (Exhibit 2). This ceiling effect reduced our statistical power to observe meaningful differences-in-changes.

We speculate that MetroHealth Care Plus's coverage and its policy of having no copays may have convinced some patients to have a recommended dilated eye examination who might not have had one if they had remained uninsured. Furthermore, Better Health's public reports and educational sessions focused attention on the importance and use of EHR-based tools to identify the need for and facilitate the completion of the examinations, making them a logical target for improvement.

Compared to people in the continuously uninsured group, MetroHealth Care Plus enrollees improved more on the diabetes outcome composite measure, as a result of greater improvement in rates of good blood pressure control. Similar to results from the Oregon experiment, our study found virtually no differences-in-

changes between the study groups for other important measures, including glycemic and lipid control and rates of obesity and tobacco use. We speculate that these negative findings are a function of both the short duration of the waiver program and the difficulty in controlling outcomes that are adversely influenced by social and behavioral determinants, especially those related to poverty.

Among MetroHealth Care Plus patients with hypertension, changes in the rate of good blood pressure control were favorable but not significantly better than changes among the comparison group (Exhibit 4). Absolute rates of good blood pressure control were comparable to national averages for enrollees in Medicaid managed care plans, as reported by National Committee for Quality Assurance,[29] and were better than the national average in 2013 (Appendix Exhibit M).[18]

These favorable results were associated with a significantly higher rate of receiving prescriptions for antihypertensive medications among MetroHealth Care Plus patients as well as higher rates of routine monitoring for renal dysfunction, compared to patients in the continuously uninsured group. Ceiling effects again reduced our power, since more than 90 percent of the members of both groups had obtained baseline blood pressure and LDL cholesterol measurements (Appendix Exhibits E and I).[18]

Our secondary analyses demonstrated significantly larger improvements in screening for or monitoring of depression among MetroHealth Care Plus enrollees who met the diabetes and hypertension criteria than among the continuously uninsured (Appendix Exhibit K).[18] The larger increase in testing for depression among MetroHealth Care Plus patients might have been related to increased acceptance of addressing mental health issues after gaining coverage, not unlike the increase in depression diagnosis among new Medicaid beneficiaries in Oregon.[3]

By contrast, we found no significant differences-in-changes between the two study groups in rates of other screening tests and tetanus vaccination. Since we examined changes in these services to determine whether selective inattention to appropriate preventive care might have declined among MetroHealth Care Plus enrollees because these standards were not publicly reported, these results are encouraging. Furthermore, higher rates of both groups at baseline met screening targets than rates reported for insured populations by the National Committee for Quality Assurance.[29] Both groups' rates of tetanus vaccination at baseline were much higher than nationwide results reported by the Centers for Disease Control and Prevention.[30]

Conclusion

We believe that the safety-net systems in this waiver program benefited from several aspects of their infrastructure (for example, patient-centered medical homes and sophisticated EHR use) and features of the program (for example, closed-panel care and health information exchange). MetroHealth Care Plus's acceptance of financial risk if the expenditure cap was exceeded also may have motivated providers to avoid unnecessary costs. Participation in a regional health improvement collaborative further prepared these safety-net systems for clinical practice transformation, accountable care, and payment reform.

These attributes of a "prepared safety net" are increasingly prevalent nationwide and deserve greater attention by state Medicaid agencies and policy makers at the federal, state, and local levels. Furthermore, despite multiple financial threats, successful safety-net organizations with these traits have been described by others.[31-35]

The one-sided financial risk in MetroHealth Care Plus contrasts with parallel positive financial incentives for better care and shared savings being tested elsewhere.[32,36,37] Regional health improvement collaboratives such as Better Health provide well-tested models in regions covering almost 40 percent of the US population.[38] The advent of these new models provides cause for optimism that the favorable results described here may underestimate the results that are possible, especially in settings with a prepared safety net and financial forces that are better aligned for better care, better health outcomes, and lower per capita costs.[39] ∎

The authors thank the leaders and health care providers of the MetroHealth System, Neighborhood Family Practice, and Care Alliance Health Center, in Cleveland, Ohio; Medical Mutual of Ohio, also in Cleveland; and the Ohio Department of Medicaid. The preparation of this article was made possible by funding from the Robert Wood Johnson Foundation and other organizations that support the Better Health Partnership, formerly Better Health Greater Cleveland.

NOTES

1 Sommers BD, Baicker K, Epstein AM. Mortality and access to care among adults after state Medicaid expansions. N Engl J Med. 2012; 367(11):1025-34.

2 Baicker K, Taubman SL, Allen HL, Bernstein M, Gruber JH, Newhouse JP, et al. The Oregon experiment—effects of Medicaid on clinical outcomes. N Engl J Med. 2013;368(18): 1713-22.

3 Taubman SL, Allen HL, Wright BJ, Baicker K, Finkelstein AN. Medicaid increases emergency-department use: evidence from Oregon's Health Insurance Experiment. Science. 2014;343(6168):263-8.

4 Centers for Medicare and Medicaid Services. Onio/MetroHealth Care Plus [Internet]. Baltimore (MD): CMS; 2013 Feb 5 [cited 2015 May 22]. Available from: http:// www.medicaid.gov/Medicaid-CHIP-Program-Information/By-Topics/ Waivers/1115/downloads/oh/oh-metrohealth-care-plus-ca.pdf

5 Kaelber DC, Waheed R, Einstadter D, Love TE, Cebul RD. Use and perceived value of health information exchange: one public healthcare system's experience. Am J Manag Care. 2013;19(10 Spec No): SP337-43.

6 Robert Wood Johnson Foundation. Aligning Forces for Quality [Internet]. Princeton (NJ): RWJF; c 2015 [cited 2015 May 14]. Available from: http://forces4quality.org/af4q-alliances-overview

7 Better Health Partnership. Data and reports [Internet]. Cleveland (OH): The Partnership; [cited 2015 June 2]. Available from: http:// betterhealthpartnership.org/data_ landing.asp. See also Notes 8 and 9.

8 Better Health Partnership. Data center: diabetes standards [Internet]. Cleveland (OH): The Partnership; [cited 2015 June 2]. Available from: http://betterhealth partnership.org/diabetes_ standards_detail.asp

9 Better Health Partnership. Data center: high blood pressure standards [Internet]. Cleveland (OH): The Partnership; [cited 2015 June 2]. Available from: http://betterhealth partnership.org/highblood pressure_standards_detail.asp

10 Cebul RD, Love TE, Jain AK, Hebert CJ. Electronic health records and quality of diabetes care. N Engl J Med. 2011;365(9):825-33.

11 In its public reports, Better Health Partnership changed its standard for good blood pressure control in patients with diabetes from <140/ 80 mmHg to <140/90 mmHg after the publication of the Eighth Joint National Committee's recommendations in 2014 (see Note 12).

12 James PA, Oparil S, Carter BL, Cushman WC, Dennison-Himmelfarb C, Handler J, et al. 2014 evidence-based guideline for the management of high blood pressure in adults: report from the panel members appointed to the Eighth Joint National Committee (JNC 8). JAMA. 2014;311(5):507-20.

13 Nolan T, Berwick DM. All-or-none measurement raises the bar on performance. JAMA. 2006;295(10): 1168-70.

14 Spitzer RL, Kroenke K, Williams JB. Validation and utility of a self-report version of PRIME-MD: the PHQ primary care study. Primary Care Evaluation of Mental Disorders. Patient Health Questionnaire. JAMA. 1999;282(18):1737-44.

15 Angrist JD, Pischke J-S. Mostly harmless econometrics: an empiricist's companion. Princeton (NJ): Princeton University Press; 2009.

16 Long JS, Ervin LH. Using heteroscedasticity consistent standard errors in the linear regression model. Am Stat. 2000;54(3):217-24.

17 Zeileis A. Econometric computing with HC and HAC covariance matrix estimators. J Stat Softw. 2004; 11(10):1-17.

18 To access the Appendix, click on the Appendix link in the box to the right of the article online.

19 Liu CW, Einstadter D, Cebul RD. Care fragmentation and emergency department use among complex patients with diabetes. Am J Manag Care. 2010;16(6):413-20.

20 Cebul RD, Rebitzer JB, Taylor LJ, Votruba ME. Organizational fragmentation and care quality in the U.S. healthcare system. J Econ Perspect. 2008;22(4):93-113.

21 Saultz JW. Defining and measuring interpersonal continuity of care. Ann Fam Med. 2003;1(3):134-43.

22 Allen H, Wright BJ, Baicker K. New Medicaid enrollees in Oregon report health care successes and challenges. Health Aff (Millwood). 2014;

33(2):292-9.

23 Roy A. Oregon study: Medicaid "had no significant effect" on health outcomes vs. being uninsured. Forbes. 2013 May 2.

24 Cannon M. Oregon study throws a stop sign in front of ObamaCare's Medicaid expansion [Internet]. Washington (DC): Cato Institute; 2013 May 3 [cited 2015 May 15]. Available from: http://www .downsizinggovernment.org/ oregon-study-throws-stop-sign-front-obamacares-medicaid-expansion

25 Cohn J. What Oregon really told us about Medicaid: a reason to rethink health care, not rethink Obamacare. New Republic [serial on the Internet]. 2013 May 13 [cited 2015 May 15]. Available from: http://www.newrepublic.com/article/113195/oregon-medicaid-study-good-bad-and-uglyy

26 Interact for Health. Rate of Ohio adults without health insurance drops [Internet]. Cincinnati (OH): Interact for Health; 2014 Aug [cited 2015 May 15]. Available from: https://www.interactforhealth.org/upl/OHIP_Uninsured_FINAL2_081214.pdf

27 Allen H, Baicker K, Finkelstein A, Taubman S, Wright BJ. What the Oregon health study can tell us about expanding Medicaid. Health Aff (Millwood). 2010;29(8):1498-506.

28 Love TE. Diabetes care and outcomes in Greater Cleveland, 2007–present

[Internet]. Cleveland (OH): Better Health Partnership; 2014 Jul 10 [cited 2015 May 15]. Figure 3. Available from: http://chrp.org//bhgcData/02_Diabetes_Care_and_Outcomes_Summer_2014.asp

29 National Committee for Quality Assurance. Improving quality and patient experience: the state of health care quality 2013 [Internet]. Washington (DC): NCQA; 2013 Oct [cited 2015 May 15]. pp. 26–33. Available from: http://www.ncqa.org/Portals/0/Newsroom/SOHC/2013/SOHC-web_version_report.pdf

30 Centers for Disease Control and Prevention. Tetanus and pertussis vaccination coverage among adults aged ≥18 years—United States, 1999 and 2008. MMWR Morb Mortal Wkly Rep. 2010;59(40):1302-6.

31 Coughlin TA, Long SK, Sheen E, Tolbert J. How five leading safety-net hospitals are preparing for the challenges and opportunities of health care reform. Health Aff (Millwood). 2012;31(8):1690-7.

32 Sandberg SF, Erikson C, Owen R, Vickery KD, Shimotsu ST, Linzer M, et al. Hennepin Health: a safety-net accountable care organization for the expanded Medicaid population. Health Aff (Millwood). 2014;33(11):1975-84.

33 Rosenbaum S, Cartwright-Smith L, Hirsh J, Mehler PS. Case studies at Denver Health: "patient dumping" in the emergency department despite EMTALA, the law that banned it.

Health Aff (Millwood). 2012;31(8):1749-56.

34 Gilman M, Adams EK, Hockenberry JM, Wilson IB, Milstein AS, Becker ER. California safety-net hospitals likely to be penalized by ACA value, readmission, and meaningful-use programs. Health Aff (Millwood). 2014;33(8):1314-22.

35 Neuhausen K, Spivey M, Kellermann AL. State politics and the fate of the safety net. N Engl J Med. 2013; 369(18):1675-7.

36 Petersen M, Muhlestein D. ACO results: what we know so far. Health Affairs Blog [blog on the Internet]. 2014 May 30 [cited 2015 May 15]. Available from: http://healthaffairs.org/blog/2014/05/30/aco-results-what-we-know-so-far/

37 Oregon Health Authority. Oregon's health system transformation: 2014 mid-year report [Internet]. Salem (OR): The Authority; 2015 Jan 14 [cited 2015 May 15]. Available from: http://www.oregon.gov/oha/Metrics/Documents/2014%20Mid-Year%20Report%20-%20Jan%20 2015.pdf

38 Cebul RD, Dade SE, Letourneau LM, Glaseroff A. Regional health improvement collaboratives needed now more than ever: program directors' perspectives. Am J Manag Care. 2012;18(6 Suppl):s112-4.

39 Berwick DM, Nolan TW, Whittington J. The Triple Aim: care, health, and cost. Health Aff (Millwood). 2008; 27(3):759-69.

Errata

WOODRUFF ET AL., 2015-0809, P. 1272 The position title for Donna Shalala should be "president of the Clinton Foundation," not "president and CEO of the Clinton Foundation." The article has been corrected online.

CEBUL ET AL., 2014-1350, P. 1123 The "factoid" on page 1123 contained an error. The phrase "continuously insured" should be "continuously uninsured." The article has been corrected online.

FAIRCHILD ET AL., 2014-1236, P. 849 In the paragraph beginning "As we have noted," the sentence beginning "All of the decrease," the city's smoking rates ticked back up in 2010, not in 2014. The article has been corrected online.

BORGHI ET AL., 2014-0808, P. 413 The acknowledgment section of this article has been revised to include acknowledgment text for one of the authors. This added text reads as follows: "Josephine Borghi is a member of the Consortium for Resilient and Responsive Health Systems (RESYST), funded by UK aid from the UK Department for International Development (DFID), and the online publication of this article was funded by RESYST/DFID. However, the views expressed and information contained in it are not necessarily those of or endorsed by the government of Norway or DFID, which can accept no responsibility for such views or information or for any reliance placed on them." The article has been corrected online.

FRED UPTON, MICHIGAN
CHAIRMAN

FRANK PALLONE, JR., NEW JERSEY
RANKING MEMBER

ONE HUNDRED FOURTEENTH CONGRESS

Congress of the United States
House of Representatives

COMMITTEE ON ENERGY AND COMMERCE
2125 RAYBURN HOUSE OFFICE BUILDING
WASHINGTON, DC 20515–6115

Majority (202) 225-2927
Minority (202) 225-3641

July 28, 2015

Ms. Victoria Wachino
Director
Center for Medicaid and CHIP Services
Centers for Medicare and Medicaid Services
7500 Security Boulevard
Baltimore, MD 21244

Dear Ms. Wachino:

Thank you for appearing before the Subcommittee on Health on July 8, 2015, to testify at the hearing entitled "Medicaid at 50: Strengthening and Sustaining the Program."

Pursuant to the Rules of the Committee on Energy and Commerce, the hearing record remains open for ten business days to permit Members to submit additional questions for the record, which are attached. The format of your responses to these questions should be as follows: (1) the name of the Member whose question you are addressing, (2) the complete text of the question you are addressing in bold, and (3) your answer to that question in plain text.

To facilitate the printing of the hearing record, please respond to these questions with a transmittal letter by the close of business on August 11, 2015. Your responses should be mailed to Graham Pittman, Legislative Clerk, Committee on Energy and Commerce, 2125 Rayburn House Office Building, Washington, D.C. 20515 and e-mailed in Word format to graham.pittman@mail.house.gov.

Thank you again for your time and effort preparing and delivering testimony before the Subcommittee.

Sincerely,

Joseph R. Pitts
Chairman
Subcommittee on Health

cc: The Honorable Gene Green, Ranking Member, Subcommittee on Health

Attachment

Ms. Wachino's response to submitted questions for the record has been retained in committee files and also is available at *http://docs.house.gov/meetings/IF/IF14/20150708/103717/HHRG-114-IF14-Wstate-WachinoV-20150708-SD002.pdf.*

FRED UPTON, MICHIGAN
CHAIRMAN

FRANK PALLONE, JR., NEW JERSEY
RANKING MEMBER

ONE HUNDRED FOURTEENTH CONGRESS

Congress of the United States
House of Representatives

COMMITTEE ON ENERGY AND COMMERCE

2125 RAYBURN HOUSE OFFICE BUILDING
WASHINGTON, DC 20515–6115

Majority (202) 225-2927
Minority (202) 225-3641

July 28, 2015

Ms. Carolyn Yocom
Director
Health Care
U.S. Government Accountability Office
441 G Street, N.W.
Washington, D.C. 20548

Dear Ms. Yocom:

Thank you for appearing before the Subcommittee on Health on July 8, 2015, to testify at the hearing entitled "Medicaid at 50: Strengthening and Sustaining the Program."

Pursuant to the Rules of the Committee on Energy and Commerce, the hearing record remains open for ten business days to permit Members to submit additional questions for the record, which are attached. The format of your responses to these questions should be as follows: (1) the name of the Member whose question you are addressing, (2) the complete text of the question you are addressing in bold, and (3) your answer to that question in plain text.

To facilitate the printing of the hearing record, please respond to these questions with a transmittal letter by the close of business on August 11, 2015. Your responses should be mailed to Graham Pittman, Legislative Clerk, Committee on Energy and Commerce, 2125 Rayburn House Office Building, Washington, D.C. 20515 and e-mailed in Word format to graham.pittman@mail.house.gov.

Thank you again for your time and effort preparing and delivering testimony before the Subcommittee.

Sincerely,

Joseph R. Pitts
Chairman
Subcommittee on Health

cc: The Honorable Gene Green, Ranking Member, Subcommittee on Health

Attachment

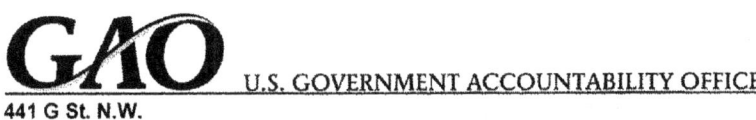

441 G St. N.W.
Washington, DC 20548

August 11, 2015

The Honorable Joseph R. Pitts
Chairman
Subcommittee on Health
Committee on Energy and Commerce
House of Representatives

Subject: Responses to Questions for the Record; Hearing Entitled *Medicaid at 50: Strengthening and Sustaining the Program*

Dear Chairman Pitts:

This letter responds to your July 28, 2015, request that we address questions for the record related to the Subcommittee's July 8th hearing on Medicaid. Our responses to the questions, which are in the enclosure, are based on our previous work and knowledge on the subjects raised by the questions.

If you have any questions about our responses to your questions or need additional information, please contact us at (202) 512-7114, iritanik@gao.gov, or yocomc@gao.gov.

Sincerely yours,

Katherine M. Iritani
Director, Health Care

Carolyn L. Yocom
Director, Health Care

Enclosure

142

The Honorable Representative Pitts

Medicaid was created to provide assistance to individuals whose income and resources are insufficient to meet the costs of necessary medical services. However, GAO has identified a number of loopholes in Medicaid financial eligibility policies that allow individuals to artificially impoverish themselves in order to qualify for Medicaid coverage of long-term care. HR 1771 is intended to address one of the loopholes GAO identified that involves the use of annuities. Can you describe the loophole GAO identified and how much money individuals are sheltering as a result of this loophole? Also, do you think that this bill would help address the problem GAO identified?

Our most recent review of Medicaid long-term care eligibility identified four main methods used by applicants to reduce their countable assets—income or resources—and qualify for Medicaid coverage.[1] In particular, married applicants may reduce their countable assets by purchasing an irrevocable and nonassignable annuity that pays potentially large amounts of income for the community spouse over a short period of time without affecting the institutionalized spouse's eligibility. A representative from one law office we spoke to in an undercover capacity suggested that the creation of an annuity can be done quickly and therefore, is a tool for last minute planning. Medicaid officials from several states said that the use of annuities for the community spouse had increased over the past few years. Officials from three states said that the increase may be a result of the passage of the Deficit Reduction Act of 2005, because it clarified how annuities for the community spouse could be set up. HR 1771 would amend Title XIX of the Social Security Act to count portions of income from annuities of a community spouse as income available to institutionalized spouses, for purposes of Medicaid eligibility. We have not made recommendations in this area, and thus cannot comment on the potential impact of HR 1771. However, the use of community spouse annuities is one approach that has been used by applicants to reduce their countable assets and qualify for Medicaid. While we did not determine by how much applicants are reducing their countable assets in this fashion, state Medicaid officials, county eligibility workers, and attorneys who provided information on the value of annuities for the community spouse reported average values ranging from $50,000 to $300,000.

The Honorable Representative Bilirakis

GAO's April 2015 report on Medicaid demonstration programs included several recommendations to CMS. Can you please provide us an update on the status of these

---

[1]See GAO, *Medicaid: Financial Characteristics of Approved Applicants and Methods Used to Reduce Assets to Qualify for Nursing Home Coverage*, GAO-14-473 (Washington, D.C.: May 22, 2014).

143

recommendations, including any actions taken by CMS and whether those actions fully address the concerns raised by your report?

In our April 2015 report, we had three recommendations regarding the Department of Health and Human Services' (HHS) demonstration approval process.[2] HHS partially agreed with one recommendation, and agreed with the two others. HHS reported to us on July 28 on certain actions the department is taking, or plans to take, in response to our recommendations. Based on information provided to date, we believe HHS has taken positive steps to respond to our recommendations, but that more actions are needed to fully respond. We will continue to examine HHS's actions and any associated documentation provided by the department. We will soon update our website with the status of HHS's responses to these recommendations, and will do so in the future as part of our annual recommendation follow-up process. Our three recommendations and HHS's responses are as follows:

- We recommended that HHS better ensure that section 1115 Medicaid demonstration approvals further Medicaid objectives by issuing criteria for assessing whether section 1115 expenditure authorities are likely to promote Medicaid objectives. HHS partially agreed with this recommendation, noting that all section 1115 Medicaid demonstrations are reviewed against "general criteria" to determine whether Medicaid objectives are met. However, HHS did not indicate plans to issue these general criteria in writing, and we maintain that more-specific guidance is needed to improve transparency.

- We also recommended that HHS ensure that the use of these criteria is documented in its approvals of demonstrations; HHS concurred with this recommendation. In July, HHS informed us of steps the department had taken since the release of our report to clarify and document in approvals the criteria used to determine whether Medicaid objectives are being met. According to HHS, the department has identified in recent approvals which of the general criteria each approved expenditure authority promotes. While this may add some transparency, we still regard HHS's general criteria as not sufficiently specific to inform stakeholders of the department's interpretation of its section 1115 authority. Moreover, these criteria are still not available as written guidance.

- Finally, we recommended that HHS take steps to ensure that its approval documentation consistently provide assurances that states will avoid duplicative spending between federal Medicaid funds for demonstrations and other federal funds available to states for the same

---

[2]See GAO, *Medicaid Demonstrations: Approval Criteria and Documentation Need to Show How Spending Furthers Medicaid Objectives*, GAO-15-239 (Washington, D.C.: April 13, 2015).

or similar purposes. HHS agreed with our recommendation and told us in July that the Centers for Medicare & Medicaid Services (CMS) will be requiring all future 1115 Medicaid demonstration approvals to include information to verify that there is no duplication of federal funding, and will work with states to document how there is no duplication of federal funding as it processes demonstration actions. We will monitor CMS's efforts in this area and will consider this recommendation to be closed if the agency implements these planned actions.

FRED UPTON, MICHIGAN
CHAIRMAN

FRANK PALLONE, JR., NEW JERSEY
RANKING MEMBER

ONE HUNDRED FOURTEENTH CONGRESS

Congress of the United States

House of Representatives

COMMITTEE ON ENERGY AND COMMERCE
2125 RAYBURN HOUSE OFFICE BUILDING
WASHINGTON, DC 20515–6115
Majority (202) 225-2927
Minority (202) 225-3641

July 28, 2015

Dr. Anne L. Schwartz
Executive Director
Medicaid and CHIP Payment and Access Commission
1800 M Street, N.W., Suite 650 South
Washington, D.C. 20036

Dear Dr. Schwartz:

Thank you for appearing before the Subcommittee on Health on July 8, 2015, to testify at the hearing entitled "Medicaid at 50: Strengthening and Sustaining the Program."

Pursuant to the Rules of the Committee on Energy and Commerce, the hearing record remains open for ten business days to permit Members to submit additional questions for the record, which are attached. The format of your responses to these questions should be as follows: (1) the name of the Member whose question you are addressing, (2) the complete text of the question you are addressing in bold, and (3) your answer to that question in plain text.

To facilitate the printing of the hearing record, please respond to these questions with a transmittal letter by the close of business on August 11, 2015. Your responses should be mailed to Graham Pittman, Legislative Clerk, Committee on Energy and Commerce, 2125 Rayburn House Office Building, Washington, D.C. 20515 and e-mailed in Word format to graham.pittman@mail.house.gov.

Thank you again for your time and effort preparing and delivering testimony before the Subcommittee.

Sincerely,

Joseph R. Pitts
Chairman
Subcommittee on Health

cc: The Honorable Gene Green, Ranking Member, Subcommittee on Health

Attachment

146

Responses to Questions for the Record
Medicaid at 50: Strengthening and Sustaining the Program
Hearing before the Health Subcommittee of the
Energy and Commerce Committee
July 8, 2015
Anne L. Schwartz, PhD
Medicaid and CHIP Payment and Access Commission

The Honorable Representative Pitts

Q1: Recently, the nonpartisan Congressional Budget Office formalized a policy to protect against conflicts of interests from their outside advisors (see: https://www.cbo. gov/about/objectivity/employee_policy). Obviously, MACPAC Commissioners are appointed because of their Medicaid and CHIP expertise and their experience representing stakeholder groups. However, given MACPAC's role as an independent source of information for Congress, similar protections against material or perceived financial or advocacy conflicts of interest may also be important for your Commissioners. In addition to the steps that GAO takes to assess potential conflicts of interest when appointing Commissioners, does MACPAC have other policies or standards for its Commissioners related to disclosing and preventing potential conflicts of interests?

    a. If so, please describe the policies or standards, including those related to the appropriate role of Commissioners in doing related but outside work or advocacy regarding Medicaid?

    b. If not, has MACPAC considered adopting conflict of interest standards? If this has been considered, please describe the Commission's plans.

A1: MACPAC's statutory language requires the Comptroller General of the U. S. to establish a system for public disclosure by members of MACPAC or financial and other potential conflicts of interest. In addition, Commission members are required to be treated as employees of Congress for the purposes of applying Title I of the Ethics in Government Act of 1978. As a result, Commissioners are required to disclose information on financial and other interests to GAO as part of the appointment process and annually thereafter. This disclosure includes information on earned income, assets and holdings, gifts and nonfederal travel reimbursement, liabilities, positions, and agreements or arrangements—requirements that are more expansive than those CBO requires of its advisors. Given the comprehensive nature of GAO's review, MACPAC has not adopted additional requirements.

Q2: MACPAC's work has reviewed some of the literature between low reimbursement rates and poor access for patients in Medicaid. Do you worry that, left unchecked, the easiest thing for legislatures to do to rein in Medicaid spending would be to cut reimbursement rates, which would have a direct negative impact on our most vulnerable patients?

A2: States have considerable flexibility under current law in the strategies they may employ to curtail Medicaid spending. These include reducing provider payments, limiting benefits, and enrolling fewer people. None of these choices are easy and all have the potential, as you note, to have a negative impact on our most vulnerable patients.

Recently, states have been engaged in a variety of activities to re-engineer the delivery system with the goal of making it more efficient while maintaining or improving quality of care or health outcomes. Over the past year, MACPAC has been examining different approaches to value-based purchasing including the use of episode-based payments in Arkansas, accountable care organizations in Minnesota, and enhanced primary care case management in Oklahoma. We also recently published findings from a review of safety-net accountable care organizations for Medicaid enrollees. In our June 2105 report, we included a chapter on the role of delivery system reform incentive payments (DSRIPs) under certain states' Section 1115 demonstrations.

While there is considerable interest in the potential of these innovations to bend the cost curve, for the most part these initiatives are still too new to have yielded clear evidence of success. Over time, we hope to get clearer answers about which approaches lead to better outcomes while moderating spending, and we look forward to keeping you informed of our work in this area.

Q3: The Commission was created five years ago. What is the most recent funding level MACPAC received, and how many staff are currently employed there?

      a.   To my knowledge, the Commission does not produce annual reports that list its staff, budget, travel expenditures, overhead, research contracts, and other spending. So, in the interest of helping the Committee better understand how MACPAC is spending taxpayer dollars, would you please make some of that data available to the Committee?

A3: MACPAC submits an annual budget justification to the House and Senate Committees on Appropriations, in accordance with their requirements. We also make that information available to the staff of MACPAC's committees of jurisdiction, including the Committee on Energy and Commerce.

In fiscal year 2015, MACPAC received an appropriation of $7. 65 million. We have requested $8. 7 million for fiscal year 2016 in order to have sufficient resources for the growing demand for technical assistance to Congressional staff and to fulfill new Congressionally mandated requirements such as our upcoming report on disproportionate share hospital (DSH) payments.

Major categories of spending include staff salaries and benefits (56 percent), external contracts for research and data analysis (21 percent), general operations (17 percent), meetings (including commissioner travel) (3 percent), and commissioner stipends (3 percent). We have a staff of 28 including analysts with experience working in state and federal governments, private sector consulting, congressional support agencies, and academia. A complete list of MACPAC staff with biographical information is included in our statutorily mandated reports and is also available on our website at https://www.macpac. gov/about-macpac/commission-staff/

MACPAC staff would be pleased to brief you or your staff on our budget and staffing, or any aspect of MACPAC operations, in more detail at your convenience.

The Honorable Representative Bilirakis

Q1: When this Committee receives a policy recommendation from MedPAC, we routinely receive the Commission's best recommendation on accompanying policies to offset the recommendation. Does MACPAC have any timeframe to adopt a similar process, providing the Committee both with recommended policy AND a recommended offset?

A1: As the transcripts of our public meetings highlight, the Commission is extremely mindful of the federal and state budget effects when making recommendations to Congress. (Note: transcripts are available at https://www. macpac. gov/public_meeting/). Indeed, consistent with MACPAC's statutory language, the Commission must examine the budget consequences of proposed recommendations. Further, recommendations must be accompanied by a report of federal and state budget implications.

I would note that, according to the Congressional Budget Office, six of the twelve recommendations MACPAC has made have been estimated to have no federal budget effect. Many of the other recommendations have been estimated to have an extremely modest budget effect—the smallest non-zero category of spending used by CBO.

The Commission will continue to consider the federal and state budget effects of recommendations they propose and consider options to mitigate budget effects, if any.

The Honorable Representative Ellmers

Q1: I'm concerned that lack of access to appropriate care often times leads to more significant costs to beneficiaries and the program, especially those with chronic conditions such as diabetes. Have you examined the impact of access to care on cost, care needs and mortality?

A1: Issues of access have been a focus of MACPAC's work since we began our work, and of course the word "access" itself is part of the Commission's name. We have examined measures of access to care for children, nonelderly adults, and populations with a disability, with results published in its annual reports to the Congress and in presentations at our public meetings. See, for example:

- Examining Access to Care in Medicaid and CHIP (March 2011) https://www. macpac. gov/publication/ch-4-examining-access-to-care-in-medicaid-and-chip/

- Examining Access and Quality in Managed Care (June 2011) https://www. macpac. gov/publication/section-e-access-and-quality-in-managed-care/

- Access to Care for Children Enrolled in Medicaid and CHIP (March 2012)

149

https://www. macpac. gov/publication/ch-2-access-to-care-for-children-enrolled-in-medicaid-or-chip/

- Access to Care for Non-Elderly Adults (March 2012)
https://www. macpac. gov/publication/section-b-access-to-care-for-non-elderly-adults/

- Access to Care for Persons with Disabilities (June 2013)
https://www. macpac. gov/publication/ch-3-access-to-care-for-persons-with-disabilities/

- Medicaid Primary Care Physician Payment Increase (June 2013)
https://www. macpac. gov/publication/ch-2-medicaid-primary-care-physician-payment-increase/

- Effects of Medicaid Coverage of Medicare Cost Sharing on Access to Care (March 2015)
https://www. macpac. gov/publication/effects-of-medicaid-coverage-of-medicare-cost-sharing-on-access-to-care/

- Provider Networks and Access: Issues for Children's Coverage (March 2015)
https://www. macpac. gov/publication/provider-networks-and-access-issues-for-childrens-coverage/

- Behavioral Health in the Medicaid Program—People, Use, and Expenditures (June 2015)
https://www. macpac. gov/publication/behavioral-health-in-the-medicaid-program%E2%80%95people-use-and-expenditures/

In general, controlling for factors such as income, age and health status, persons enrolled in Medicaid do not differ substantially from those with private insurance in their use of health services. Medicaid enrollees have better access to medical care than those without health insurance, again controlling for many sociodemographic characteristics. Medicaid enrollees use more emergency room visits and have longer wait times than those who are privately insured, but fewer concerns over costs of care. After accounting for differing enrollee characteristics, children with Medicaid or CHIP and those with employer-sponsored insurance report similar rates of delayed medical care.

Because Medicaid populations are on average poorer and less healthy than privately insured populations, it is difficult to independently assess the effect of having Medicaid on health outcomes. Moreover, lack of available data make it difficult to assess the relationship between use of specific services and health outcomes associated with use of those services.

Looking at access to care at the national level does not answer the question of whether specific groups of Medicaid enrollees face barriers to accessing specific services. MACPAC's work plan for its 2016 reports includes additional analysis of access to care for specific populations, including children, nonelderly adults, older adults, and persons with disabilities. We are particularly interested in learning whether Medicaid beneficiaries are using recommended services that have been shown to improve health outcomes, such as preventive screenings, dental care, and behavioral health care. We are also interested in learning how such use compares to privately insured persons in similar income and age groups. The Commission is also specifically interested in barriers to treatment for persons with behavioral health conditions and whether there are ways to organize the delivery of care, such as programs to integrate mental health and medical care, which have been shown to reduce expenditures and provide better outcomes.

Q2: Have you examined the published evidence of Medicaid patient access barriers to podiatrists and the experience of state Medicaid programs that have ensured access to podiatrists?

A2: States may, but are not required, to provide podiatry services under Medicaid programs. In addition, such services may be limited to specific populations or specific conditions. For example, in California, podiatry services are limited to pregnant women and institutionalized adults. Other limitations vary by type of service and include limits on the number of services covered per month (KFF 2015). In the state of Nevada, Medicaid only cover podiatry services for dually eligible Medicare and Medicaid enrollees and children who are referred based on screening (Nevada Department of Health and Human Services 2015).

Although MACPAC has not independently analyzed how coverage of podiatry services affects outcomes and costs, we are familiar with several recent studies demonstrating that podiatry services may reduce subsequent morbidity and mortality, particularly among persons with diabetes. A 2011study found that patients who visited a podiatric physician had $13,474 lower costs in commercial plans and $3,624 lower costs in Medicare plans during two-year follow-up (Carls et al. 2011). A study of Medicaid enrollee costs before and after the podiatric benefit was removed in the Arizona Medicaid program in 2009 found an increase in hospitalizations and costs among diabetic enrollees (Skrepnek et al. 2014).

References

Carls G. S. , T.B. Gibson, V.R. Driver, et al. 2011. The economic value of specialized lower-extremity medical care by podiatric physicians in the treatment of diabetic foot ulcers. *Journal of the American Podiatric Medical Association* 101, no. 2: 93–115. http://www. apma. org/files/FileDownloads/TR-JAPMA-Article. pdf

The Henry J. Kaiser Family Foundation (KFF). 2015. Medicaid benefits: Podiatrist services. *State Health Facts.* http://kff. org/medicaid/state-indicator/podiatrist-services/.

Nevada Department of Health and Human Services. 2015. Nevada provider type 21 billing guide. Carson City, Nevada: Nevada Department of Health and Human Services. https://www. medicaid. nv. gov/Downloads/provider/NV_BillingGuidelines_PT21. pdf

Skrepnek G.H., J.L. Mills, and D.G. Armstrong. 2014. Foot-in-wallet disease: Tripped up by "cost-saving" reductions? *Diabetes Care* 37: e196–e197. http://care.diabetesjournals.org/content/37/9/e196.full.pdf

www.ingramcontent.com/pod-product-compliance
Lightning Source LLC
Chambersburg PA
CBHW081126170526

45165CB00008B/2570